AF327982

World Clinics in Ophthalmology

Recent Trends in Cataract Management

Volume 1

Editors:

Arnaldo Espaillat Matos, MD

Amar Agarwal, MS, FRCS, FRC. Ophth.

Richard Lindstrom, MD

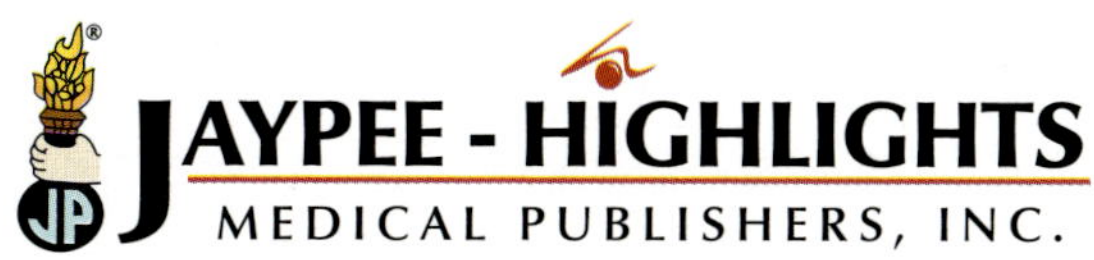

JAYPEE - HIGHLIGHTS
MEDICAL PUBLISHERS, INC.

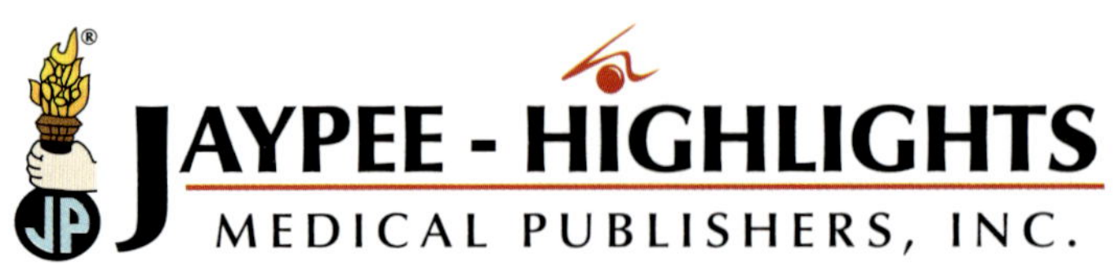

An Editorial Branch of Jaypee Brothers Medical Publishers (P) Ltd.

PRODUCTION
Editor-in-Chief: Samuel Boyd, MD
Production Director: Kayra Mejia
Chief, Digital Composition: Laura Duran, Erick Navarro
Art Director: Eduardo Chandeck
International Communications: Joyce Ortega

MARKETING
Director Sales & Marketing Latin America: Srinivas Chaubey
Customer Service: Miroslava Bonilla
Sales Manager: Tomas Martinez

World Clinics in Ophthalmology -
Recent Trends in Cataract Management

Editors: Arnaldo Espaillat Matos, MD; Amar Agarwal, MS, FRCS, FRC. Ophth.; Richard Lindstrom, MD

ISSN 2224-1353

Published for: Jaypee - Highlights Medical Publishers, Inc.
City of Knowledge
International Technopark, Bldg. 237
Gaillard Highway, Clayton
Panama Rep. of Panama

Phone: (507) 301-0496 / 97 - Fax: (507) 301-0499
E-mail: cservice@jphmedical.com
Worldwide Web: www.jphmedical.com

Acknowledgment

Cataract surgery techniques have as their goal the complete elimination of the need for a post cataract surgery spectacle whether by means of multifocal IOLs, accommodative IOLs, toric IOLs, femtosecond laser technology, and, last but not least, capsular bag refilling techniques the latter regarded by the cataract/refractive surgeon as the holy grail of surgical goals.

The main aim of this Volume is to answer the questions most patients ask about cataracts, using non-technical language and a supportive tone, including what a cataract is, how it forms, what the various types of surgery entail and when each is appropriate, and what to expect in the recovery stages. The book covers new advances in diagnosis and treatments.

Our first major acknowledgement is to the Contributing Authors who have worked diligently in presenting their initial concepts to final page proofs in their interesting chapters. We are also grateful and thank for the wonderful support we received from the staff at Jaypee Highlights Medical Publishers, who played a key role in bringing this Volume to a successful conclusion.

The Editors

Foreword

Since Sir Harold Ridley's first intraocular lens implantation in 1949, intraocular lens technology has developed exponentially. As a result, intraocular lens implantation has become the most successful and most widely performed surgery in human organ transplantation in the modern medical era. At the same time, ophthalmologists have, over the past 40 years, seen a dramatic renaissance in cataract surgery technique. Furthermore, having achieved the initial goal of primary aphakic correction, the evolving technology now permits the correction of astigmatism, higher order aberrations and even presbyopia, the latter once considered to be an unattainable dream.

Following ICCE and ECCE techniques, the advent of Kelman's phacoemulsification technology in the early 1970's was a paradigm shift in cataract implant technique. It encouraged the development and refinement of cataract removal and intraocular lens technology so that along with small incision cataract surgery, a new standard of modern cataract surgery now exists.

Consequently, postoperative inflammation and severe ocular complications have been minimized. A high quality of vision, once achieved rarely and then with difficulty, has now become an expected outcome. At the same time, novel materials and designs of IOLs have been developed that provide improved biocompatibility and reduce the late capsular opacification that can threaten post operative visual acuity.

Today, refractive lens surgery techniques have as their goal the complete elimination of the need for a post cataract surgery spectacle whether by means of multifocal IOLs, accommodative IOLs, toric IOLs, femtosecond laser technology, and, last but not least, capsular bag refilling techniques, the latter regarded by the cataract/refractive surgeon as the holy grail of surgical goals.

These procedures, along with the currently available attractive technological advances of reproductive medicine using iPS cells, have created for the cataract/refractive surgical investigator bent on solving presbyopia a never more exciting time full of the potential for novel possibilities derived from applying these and other technologies.

Drs. Agarwal, Espaillat and Lindstrom have compiled a superb comprehensive book that addresses all the components of refractive lens surgery by including international experts whose expertise have resulted in the recent advances refractive lens surgery. This book will definitely provide both the experienced as well as the novice cataract surgeon, the rationale for current refractive lens surgery that will be of benefit to their patients. The dramatic changes in ophthalmological technology that this cutting edge book presents will, without doubt, act as the nidus in the near future for further editions containing additional technological breakthroughs that, I hope, this book will be of help to further.

Dr. Okihiro Nishi
Professor and Head
Nishi Eye Hospital,
Nakamichi, Higashinari-Ku,
Osaka, Japan

Editors

Arnaldo Espaillat Matos, MD
Medical Director
Instituto Espaillat Cabral
Santo Domingo, Dominican Republic

Amar Agarwal, MS, FRCS, FRC. Ophth.
Eye Research Centre & Dr. Agarwal's Group of Eye Hospitals
Chennai, Bangalore, Trichy, Jaipur, Salem,
Kerala, India

Richard Lindstrom, MD
Founder & Attending Surgeon,
Minnesota Eye Consultants, P.A.
Adjunct Professor Emeritus at the
Department of Ophthalmology, University of Minnesota,
Minnesota, USA

Contributors

Amar Agarwal, MS, FRCS, FRC. Ophth.
Eye Research Centre & Dr. Agarwal's Group of Eye Hospitals
Chennai, Bangalore, Trichy, Jaipur, Salem,
Kerala, India

Athiya Agarwal, MD, FRSH, DO
Eye Research Centre & Dr. Agarwal's Group of Eye Hospitals
Chennai, Bangalore, Trichy, Jaipur, Salem,
Kerala, India

Sunita Agarwal, MS, FSVH, DO
Eye Research Centre & Dr. Agarwal's Group of Eye Hospitals
Chennai, Bangalore, Trichy, Jaipur, Salem,
Kerala, India

Jorge L. Alio, MD, PhD
Vissum - Instituto Oftalmológico Alicante,
Refractive Surgery and Cornea Department,
Miguel Hernández University, Medical School,
Alicante, Spain

Shaloo Bageja, MS
Consultant, Department of Ophthalmology
Sir Gangaram Hospital
Rajender Nagar
New Delhi, India

Samuel Boyd, MD
Director, Laser Section, and Associate Director,
Clinica Boyd - Ophthalmology Center
Panama, Rep. of Panama

Ahmed Galal, MD, PhD
Vissum - Instituto Oftalmológico Alicante,
Refractive Surgery and Cornea Department,
Miguel Hernández University, Medical School,
Alicante, Spain

AK Grover, MD, FRCS
Chairman, Department of Ophthalmology
Sir Gangaram Hospital
Rajender Nagar
New Delhi, India

Robert M. Kershner, MD, MS, FACS
Professor III and Chairman, Department of Ophthalmic Medical Technology,
Palm Beach State College, BioScience Technology Center,
Palm Beach Gardens, Florida, USA
Consulting Surgeon, Eye Laser Consulting, Boston, Massachusetts, USA

Flavio Koji Narazaki, MD
Cataract Institute (INCAT)
Vision Institute
Department of Ophthalmology,
Sao Paulo Federal University,
Brazil

Lincoln Lemes Freitas, MD
Director, Cataract Institute (INCAT)
Vision Institute
Department of Ophthalmology,
Sao Paulo Federal University,
Brazil

Jose-Luis Rodriguez Prats, MD
Vissum - Instituto Oftalmológico Alicante,
Refractive Surgery and Cornea Department,
Miguel Hernández University, Medical School,
Alicante, Spain

George O. Waring IV, MD
Director of Refractive Surgery, Storm Eye Institute;
Assistant Professor of Ophthalmology,
Medical University of South Carolina, Charleston, SC;
Medical Director, Magill Vision Center; Mt. Pleasant,
South Carolina, United States

World Clinics in Ophthalmology
Recent Trends in Cataract Management
Volume 1

Contents

Samuel Boyd, MD

1 Preoperative Selection for Cataract Surgery

To date there is no established medical treatment for the prevention or treatment of cataract formation and thus the treatment of cataracts remains surgical. Contrary to the commonly held belief that cataracts must reach a certain degree of density or become "ripe" prior to considering cataract surgery, today the crystalline lens can be removed at virtually any stage.

Role of Quality of Life

Cataract/IOL surgery improves quality of life better than any other medical procedure known to mankind. Cataract surgery is indicated when the patient's quality of life is being affected by visual impairment, when there is a diminution in vision if the patient is exposed to light or at night, and when the preoperative evaluation indicates that the potential for restoration of sight is good. How much a patient's quality of life is impaired from a cataract is relative, varying with the patient's occupation and age.[1] The key factor is not to wait until a nuclear cataract becomes hard. With time, the lens fiber density becomes a hard nuclear brunescent cataract. Even with most modern phacoemulsification techniques sometimes it may become difficult to perform surgery if the lens becomes extremely dense or brunescent.

Waiting too long may require that the surgeon operate on dense nuclear cataracts, which increases the risk of posterior capsule tears, whether we perform planned extracapsular, SICS *(Small Incision Cataract Surgery)* or a phacoemulsification **(Figure 1)**. This complication may lead to other rather serious problems

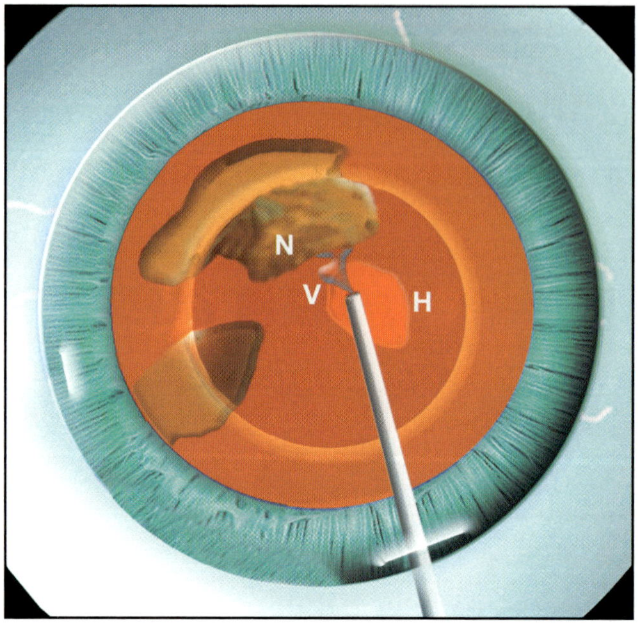

Figure 1: Complications with Posterior Capsule Rupture. A disruption of the posterior capsule (H) is a serious intraoperative complication. If no immediate action is taken, luxation of nucleus material (N) to the vitreous and retina may occur. If vitreous prolapse is present and it mixes with nucleus fragments, the vitreous should be addressed first. To solve this complication the surgeon must stop the maneuvers of nucleus removal. Proceed immediately to inject viscoelastic (V) under the nucleus fragments to push the vitreous and lens fragments away from the posterior capsule tear. In this figure, only a "trickle" of viscoelastic (V) is seen between the tear and the nucleus fragments. The rest of the viscoelastic is underneath the nucleus attempting to push it away from the tear. At this time it is indicated to perform a well controlled anterior "dry vitrectomy" in which no infusion is used or one with a very low flow system. If abundant nuclear material still remains after these measures are taken, the surgeon may choose between converting to ECCE or very carefully continuing with phacoemulsification decreasing significantly the power, flow and vacuum settings. It depends on the surgeon's experience. (Art from Jaypee Highlights)

such as dislocated nucleus, retinal detachment, macular edema, bullous keratopathy and inflammation. [2]

The Role of Visual Acuity

There are very few strict criteria for recommending cataract surgery. In the United States, however, many professional review organizations have indicated that the reduction of Snellen distance acuity to 20/40 or worse as a result of cataract is sufficient indication in and of itself for cataract surgery. This is generally the minimum standard for driving. In some of the advanced, developed countries, being unable to obtain a driver's license may seriously affect a person's life because he/she may be disqualified to drive to the market or shop to purchase food and other materials essential to daily existence. However, in many cases surgery may be indicated without reduction of visual acuity to the level of 20/40 if the patient has difficulty performing activities of daily living.[3] Because patients have varying occupational and recreational needs, some patients may need cataract surgery prior to having their vision reduced to 20/40 by standard tests.

In addition, near vision in some cases may be compromised more than distance acuity particularly in the case of central posterior subcapsular cataracts. The trend toward early removal of cataract offers the advantage of operating on a younger age group, many of whom are still productive members of society.

Their need for early return to their usual lifestyle is extremely important. The older population, often living alone, also benefits from early visual recovery. These high expectations and needs require that the ophthalmic surgeon perform superior surgery to obtain excellent postoperative visual acuity and early visual rehabilitation.

As emphasized by Richard Lindstrom, symptoms of cataracts include complaints of a yellowing of vision, glare, halos, decreased night vision, and generally blurred vision in adults. Nuclear sclerosis which is a typical form of age-related cataracts may also induce a myopic shift and patients may give a history of having changed their glasses several times within a short period of time. In children cataracts may present as leukocoria and may result in strabismus and/or amblyopia if not treated promptly.

Details of the Preoperative Evaluation

A patient's preoperative evaluation can help avoid any condition that will delay or eliminate the promised or anticipated postoperative result. Surgeons should review a patient's medical and surgical history and be careful with patients who have diabetes or collagen vascular or autoimmune disease. Other concerns include previous ocular or corneal surgery and previous and existing ophthalmic conditions, such as macular degeneration, glaucoma, strabismus, amblyopia, and dry eye.[4]

Patients who wear soft contact lenses should discontinue lens wear at least 2 weeks before examination, and patients who wear hard or rigid gas-permeable (RGP) lenses should discontinue lens wear at least 3 weeks before examination for reliable keratometry readings in the preoperative evaluation. A stable ocular surface with reliable keratometry readings is desired. Hard contact or RGP lens wearers should have keratometry readings taken at 1-week intervals, and the last two readings must not differ by > 0.5 D.

In the preoperative examination, surgeons should also determine eye dominance, visual acuity, and refraction. The keratometer must be calibrated, and surgeons should perform a pupillary examination, measuring in bright and dim light illumination. Corneal topography and/or Pentacam exam is necessary for all patients to rule out keratoconus or any other abnormality, to check ocular surface quality, and to plan for astigmatism management.

Surgeons should also confirm agreement between the topographic and keratometric cylinder; otherwise, it`s recommended for surgeons to proceed carefully and repeat measurements. Astigmatism is not always reflected on keratometry readings, however. Topography thus may be helpful in diagnosing irregular astigmatism.

Contrast Sensitivity and Glare Disability

In evaluating a patient with cataract and in the process of deciding when that person requires cataract/IOL surgery, it is fundamental to keep always in mind that standard Snellen acuity measurements do not give any information with regard to symptoms of disabling glare.[5] As a matter of fact, very good visual acuity with the Snellen chart in the physician's examining room may lead the ophthalmologist to making the wrong decision and recommendations unless he or she takes other factors into consideration. In later years, we have become increasingly aware that diminished contrast sensitivity which interferes with sharp vision under different color backgrounds or target luminance, is an essential element of sight and a highly limiting factor in the presence of cataract. This is perceived by the patient for example when he or she is unable to read a computer screen at the airport if the background is light blue and the print is light yellow even though visual acuity in the physician's refracting lane was 20/30 or 20/25.

These are additional very important issues in determining when the cataract should be removed. For many years this judgment has been based on Snellen visual acuity. But a patient can score quite well on Snellen acuity while suffering in real life. Posterior subcapsular cataracts are notorious for interfering with reading, even when distance vision is good, and may induce a great deal of glare. Snellen acuity may be 20/20 or 20/25, but against oncoming headlights while driving at night, for instance, the glare may diminish the functional vision to 20/100 or even 20/200.

People with nuclear sclerosis, the most common form of cataract, tend to be bothered by decreased contrast sensitivity rather than glare. Although glare disability and contrast sensitivity are distinctly different, the terms often are erroneously interchanged. The testing characteristics of each, however, may overlap, and a reduction in one function often leads to a diminution in the other, further adding to the confusion of their differences.[5] As clarified by Samuel Masket, glare disability is a light-induced visual symptom. Contrast sensitivity testing is a means of vision analysis, analogous to a markedly expanded form of Snellen acuity evaluation at varied amounts of target luminance.

Contrast Sensitivity Characteristics

Like audiometry, which measures the sensitivity of the hearing apparatus to stimuli at different audio frequencies, contrast sensitivity analysis determines the ability of the visual system to perceive objects of differing contrasts as well as sizes. A patient who has a reduction in contrast sensitivity might perceive the small, highly contrasted targets on a Snellen test line but be incapable of identifying larger objects at reduced contrast. There are alterations in the visual system that can cause visual loss not detected by the determination of Snellen visual acuity but may be evaluated by testing of contrast sensitivity function. This is unlike disabling glare, which determines the effect of extraneous light on visual performance. Contrast sensitivity evaluation is a measurement of the resolving power of the eye at varied contrasts between image and background.

Relation of Glare to Type of Cataract

Neumann et al. have determined that nuclear cataract is more likely to be associated with nighttime glare disability, while cortical cataract formation is associated with daylight glare, and posterior subcapsular cataracts may induce glare disability associated with bright, direct sunlight or bright central light sources. Cortical cataracts seem more likely to cause glare symptoms than nuclear cataracts. Masket points out that frequently, patients with dense central posterior subcapsular cataracts frequently retain excellent distance Snellen acuity as measured in the refracting lane, yet they perform poorly on any of the available glare testing devices. Such patients may have severely lower visual function during daylight driving although they do well with the Snellen acuity chart. In essence, the Snellen chart evaluates quantity of vision. Contrast sensitivity tests evaluate quantity and quality of vision.

Preoperative Considerations

In addition to determining visual acuity by the Snellen chart, contrast sensitivity and glare disability testing as outlined, all patients with cataracts should have a thorough history taken including any systemic or ocular medications being used and any systemic disease for which they receive treatment.[6] A family history is also included. The ophthalmologic examination should include intraocular pressure (IOP) measurements, keratometry, pupil exam, routine motility

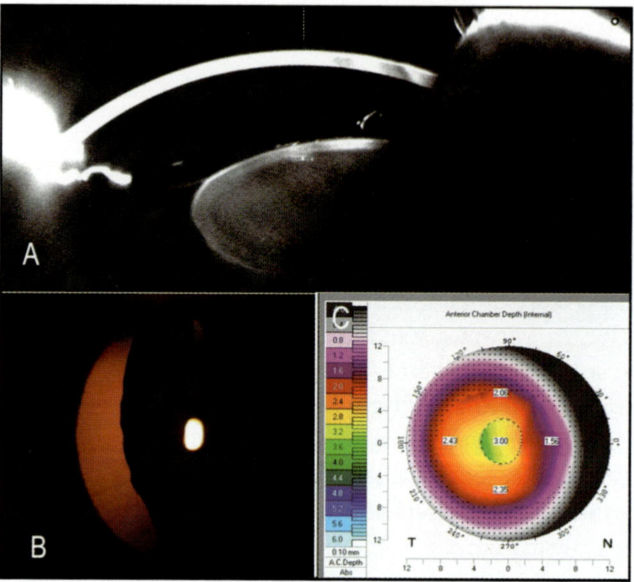

Figure 2: Scheimpflug image of lens sub-luxation (A) in a case referred for evaluation of astigmatism and suspicious of ectasia. Note the biomicroscopic findings (B) and the anterior chamber asymmetry in the depth (C).

testing, and dilated slit-lamp and funduscopic examinations including indirect ophthalmoscopy to examine the central and peripheral retina. Ancillary testing such as visual fields, topography or Pentacam, specular microscopy for endothelial cell counts, and fluorescein angiography should be considered in selected cases **(Figure 2)**. There are many causes for decreased vision and, especially in older patients, these causes may exist concurrently. Age-related macular degeneration is possibly the most important and difficult to detect because of the existing opacity of the cataract.[7]

Additional Tests

Adequate assessment for dry eye is also important and can be performed using slit lamp examination. It is important to consider that visual recovery may be delayed if the condition is not treated. A healthy ocular surface is also necessary to obtain reliable keratometry readings. Preoperative evaluation of precorneal tear film and ocular surface is necessary and can be accomplished using Schirmer's test, fluorescein staining, or vital dyes.

Slit lamp examination will allow surgeons to identify patients with pseudoexfoliation syndrome or corneal guttata or Fuchs' dystrophy. Patients with corneal guttata or Fuchs' dystrophy are at risk of reduced visual function, disease progression, and postoperative corneal edema.

Evaluation of Macular Function

Some of the main preoperative tests to determine central visual acuity still are: 1) the Potential Visual Acuity Meter (PAM) and 2) the Super Pinhole. They permit evaluation of the macular function in patients in whom examination of the macula is difficult due to media opacities.

They are more useful when they are integrated into the total evaluation of the patient. One of the major problems that all of us confront as clinical ophthalmologists is that of patients with cataracts who correct to 20/100 or 20/200 and on whom we are planning to operate but cannot see the fundus, particularly the macula.[8] This is aggravated when the patient has a few old small corneal opacities. The ever-present question is: what is the visual prognosis if we operate, either by a cataract extraction or combined with a corneal transplant?

What can we anticipate for the patient or his/her family about future, postoperative vision even if we do not have any significant operative or postoperative complications? Ultrasonography and clinical tests will give us only a partial and limited answer. Since we cannot see clearly the state of the macula or papilla, we are limited as to the prognosis. Sometimes we have the pleasant surprise of obtaining more vision postoperatively than we predicted; in other cases, we face the unpleasant reality of finding macular degeneration or other lesions in the macula or optic nerve that result in poor central vision in spite of a beautifully performed operation.

Any well trained ophthalmologist can diagnose major lesions of the optic nerve or retina preoperatively. The major problem is with the subtle lesions that nevertheless limit the patient's capacity to read or distinguish clear images at distance postoperatively **(Figure 3)**.

The Importance of Pre-Op Fundus Exam

Thorough peripheral retinal examination should be done before cataract extraction. We are all proud to be first class clinical ophthalmologists and not think of cataract surgery only as a mechanical, technical procedure.[9] As patients live longer, they are apt to have more preoperative diseases sometimes difficult to diagnose unless we are on the alert for them.

Because the patient with an even moderate degree of cataract has reduced clarity of vision, it is easily possible that recent abnormalities may not have been observed or reported by the patient. This is particularly the case with retinal diseases.

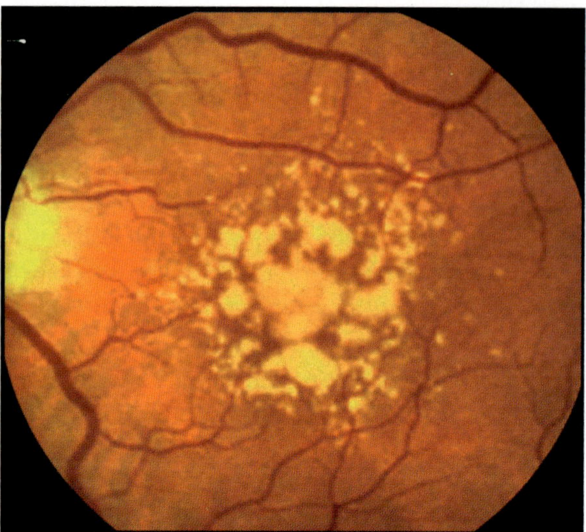

Figure 3: Soft drusen are dome-shaped coalescence elevations, containing proteins and lipofuscin.

Cataract Surgery in Diabetic Patients

Because of the increasing importance of diabetic retinopathy, both in incidence and severity, we provide special emphasis to this disease in considering cataract surgery in complex cases. Cataract and retinovascular complications often co-exist in diabetic patients.

The combination can present problems in determining the cause of decreased vision. Cataract surgery can also result in rapid progression of diabetic retinopathy that may need treatment with photocoagulation **(Figure 4)**.

Diabetic patients are very predisposed to developing cataracts. This is especially true of younger diabetic patients, who are also highly predisposed to developing diabetic retinopathy (diabetes Type I). In a series of diabetic retinopathy and maculopathy patients 15 years after laser treatment, only 22% of the eyes maintained clear lenses.

Cataracts will often form following vitrectomy surgery for diabetic retinopathy. Rarely retinopathy can cause cataracts. An example would be prolonged vitreous cavity hemorrhage that results in a partial opacification of the lens. (Very high risk proliferative diabetic retinopathy).

Cataract Surgery in Patients with Uveitis

Rubens Belfort Jr., in Sao Paulo, Brazil has conducted extensive research on these patients. Cataracts develop frequently in patients with uveitis, either as a

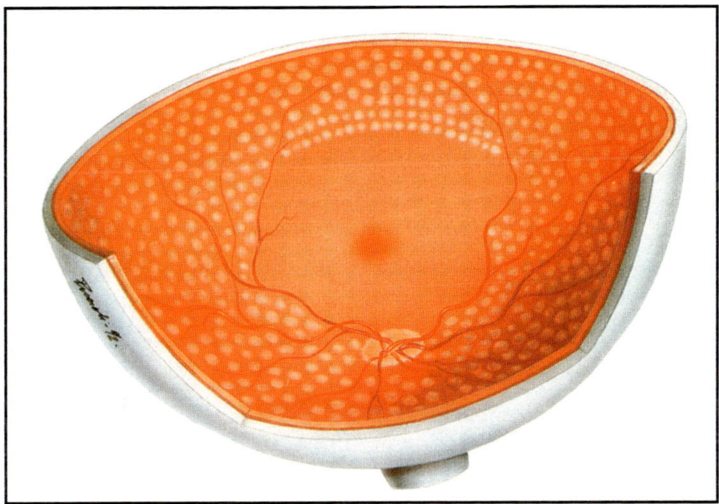

Figure 4: Panretinal Laser Photocoagulation Before Cataract Surgery. In treating diabetic retinopathy, panretinal photoco- agulation covers all of the periphery and mid-periphery of the retina from the ora serrata to the vascular arcades, sparing only the posterior pole. (Photo courtesy of Prof. Rosario Brancato, M.D., from Milan, Italy, reproduced from "Practical Guide to Laser Photocoagulation", Italian Edition by Brancato, Coscas and Lumbroso, published by SIFI.)

result of inflammation, the treatment of inflammation or both. There has been much controversy as to what to do, how to do it and when to operate in patients with cataract and uveitis, and what type of intraocular lenses should be implanted in these patients.

Professor Rubens Belfort Jr. considers that uveitis is one of the last categories for which surgeons have advised «don't do it» when cataract surgery is considered. Cataract surgery has been regarded as contraindicated because of the initial bad results with intraocular lenses (IOLs) in patients with uveitis. There was concern about superimposing IOL implantation, with the inflammation which used to accompany it in many cases, on a seriously compromised and already inflamed eye. This concept has now changed. The development of current techniques for small incision cataract surgery, new types of IOLs, and advances in the medical management of patients with uveitis have changed the prognosis. The change is fortunate because cataracts are the major cause of loss of vision in patients with chronic uveitis. Moreover, cataracts are potentially dangerous for patients with uveitis because they interfere with visualization of the fundus, denying the ophthalmologist the opportunity to identify macular lesions and to treat them adequately. When these patients finally undergo long-postponed surgery, usually with good anatomic success, central vision may not be recovered because of irreversible macular damage that had developed from chronic cystoid macular edema (Fortunately, today we have a vast group of intraocular medications that may help these patients to recover from these uncertain retinal pathologies). Therefore it is critical for both the surgeon and the patient with uveitis to realize there is another reason for cataract surgery in addition to improving vision as much as possible. Removal of the cataract enables the ophthalmologist to examine and treat the macula in order to stabilize the previous damage.

Intraocular Lenses

Proper patient selection is the first important step to ensure the type of IOL you`ll recommend to your patients. Successful multifocal IOL implantation can greatly increase the number of satisfied patients since they will improve distance, intermediate and near vision **(Figure 5)**.

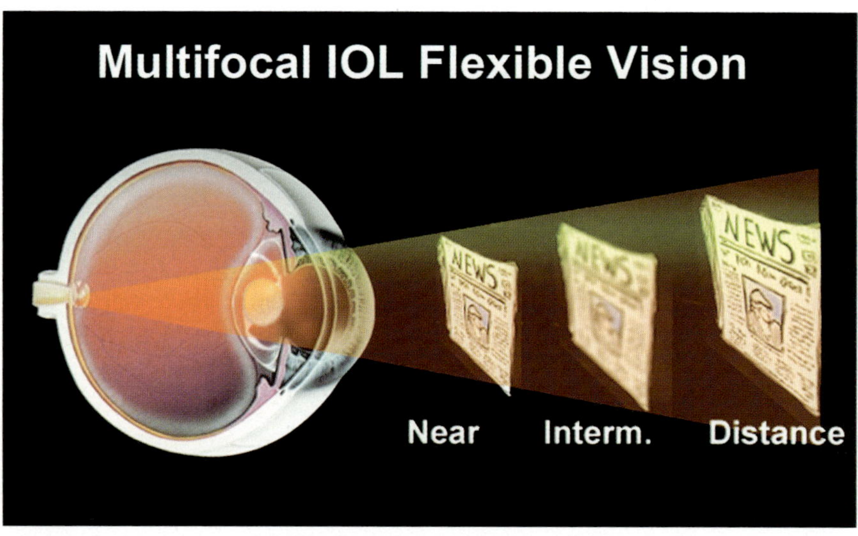

Figure 5: Multifocal IOL. By implanting multifocal IOLs, and by taking a few additional steps, you can correct ametropia and presbyopia at the same time and give an intermediate vision which these patients lack.

Patient Needs and Expectations

Preoperatively, the surgeon should discuss the option of multifocal IOLs with patients with cataracts. The surgeon should interact with patients to develop a relationship and to determine their vision needs. In addition, surgeons must educate patients preoperatively so they know what outcomes to expect, increasing the likelihood of patient satisfaction. Patients are more likely to tolerate expected outcomes than unanticipated outcomes.[10] Furthermore, surgeons must understand the vision demands of each patient and should take time to learn about each patient's daily activities, such as night driving habits, computer use, reading habits, and sports or performance activities. For example, a night-time taxi driver in New York City may look at point sources of light all night. An IOL that could create glare, therefore, is not an appropriate option for this patient **(Figure 6)**.

In addition to evaluating a patient's vision needs, surgeons should also determine whether a patient is tolerant or demanding. Evaluating the patient's traits will greatly affect the surgeon's management of patient expectations.

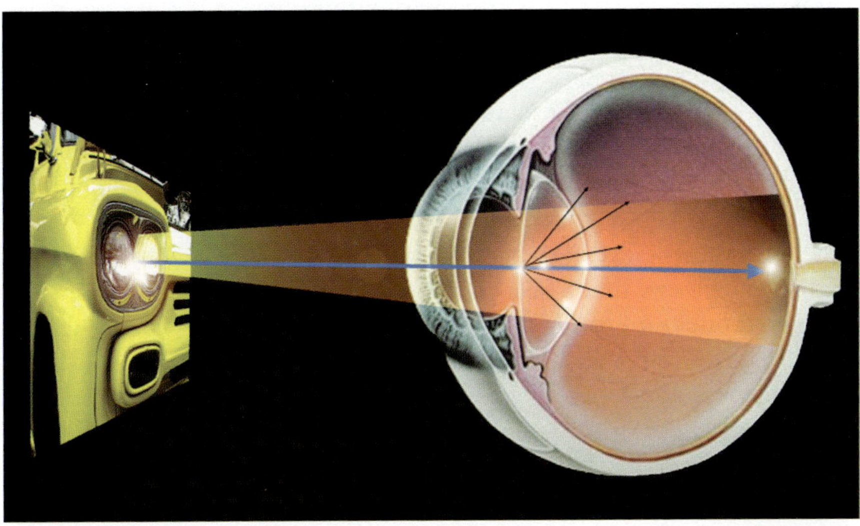

Figure 6: Night's Disadvantages. Optical side effects of multifocal IOLs should not be overemphasized. Fortunately, the new generation of multizone refractive lenses produces fewer of these phenomena. We must be aware that photic phenomena are only a night condition and also tend to regress after a time.

Stress Functional Vision

The goal of implanting a multifocal IOL in patients is to reduce dependence on glasses. In the preoperative discussion, surgeons should explain to patients that visual outcomes might not be as clear as outcomes with glasses, but I believe patients will be happy when provided with the best possible distance, intermediate, and near vision.

With reasonable expectations, multifocal's strengths can be emphasized. In clinical experience, these IOL offers patients excellent distance vision specially in bright light, reading vision, and intermediate vision for many of today's functional tasks, such as using a computer.

Intermediate vision is also necessary to accomplish other tasks, such as serving and eating food, looking at a wristwatch or dashboard gauges, and dialing on a cellular phone, among others.

The Ideal Patient

Patients who have an acceptance of realistic goals and motivation to reduce dependence on glasses are favorable candidates for multifocal IOLs. Motivated patients are more willing than other patients to tolerate the process of reducing dependence on glasses with multifocal IOL implantation and to recognize that some time is required to adapt to the new visual system.

Patients with cataracts, with or without presbyopia, are also ideal. In addition, patients who are candidates for bilateral implantation, as well as patients with hyperopia, are preferred.

The ideal patient will also understand that loss of contrast is possible. Surgeons should explain that in addition to possible contrast loss, patients may experience glare or halos and that glasses may be necessary for work requiring prolonged near vision.

Patient acceptance of the process with multifocal IOL implantation also relies on the knowledge that a second procedure may be necessary. I inform patients that about one third of all patients will require another procedure to treat residual spherical error or residual astigmatism.

Surgeons should carefully consider patients who have unrealistic expectations and who are overly critical, such as patients who complain of significant glare with contact lenses. Patients with night-time occupations, as well as pilots, should also be carefully considered.

Previous refractive surgery or the potential for progressive keratoconus or age-related macular degeneration may also be concerns for multifocal IOL implantation.

Editorial Comment

Considering that cataract surgery entails a significant impact on the quality of life, the correct selection of the patient that may require this procedure is very important. Evaluation of the individual's lifestyle and specific visual needs provides valuable orientation as to when the surgery should be performed. The patient's general and ocular medical history, the assessment of the quantity and quality of his/her vision, a thorough ophthalmological examination and the use of the appropriate diagnostic technology, will yield the necessary information for the visual prognosis and the planning of the surgery.

Arnaldo Espaillat, MD

References

1. Boyd, BF.: Cataract Surgery in Diabetic Patients. World Atlas Series of Ophthalmic Surgery. In: Highlights of Ophthalmology, Vol. IV, 1999; 9:153-54.
2. Boyd, BF.: Undergoing cataract surgery with a master surgeon: A personal experience. Highlights of Ophthalm. Journal, Vol. 27, N° 1, 1999; 2-3.
3. Charlton, Judie: Cataract surgery and lens implantation. Editorial Overview, Current Opinion in Ophthalmology, 2000, 11:1-2.
4. Fine, IH.: Cataract surgical problem: Consultation section. J Cataract Refractive Surg, 1997; 23:704.
5. Gimbel, HV., Anderson Penno, EE: Cataracts: Pathogenesis and treatment. Canadian Journal of Clinical Medicine, September 1998.
6. Gimbel HV., Basti S., Ferensowicz MA., DeBroff BM: Results of bilateral cataract extraction with posterior chamber intraocular lens implantation in children. Ophthalmology, 1997; 104:1737-1743.
7. John K., Fenzl R.: Preoperative Workup. Cataract Surgery: The State of the Art. Edited by Gills, JP.Slack; 1998; 1:1-8.
8. Lacava, AC., Caballero, JC., Medeiros, OA., Centurion, V.: Biometria no alto miope. Rev Bras de Oft. 1995; 54:619-622.
9. Masket S.: Preoperative evaluation of the patient with visually significant cataract. Atlas of Cataract Surgery, Edited by Masket S. & Crandall AS. In: Martin Dunitz Ltd., 1999, 1:3-5.
10. Neumann D., Weissmann OD., Isenberg SJ., et al: The effectiveness of daily wear contact lenses for correction of infantile aphakia. Arch Ophthalmol. 1993; 111:927-9.

2 | Optimizing Refractive Outcome: Surgical Correction of Astigmatism in Cataract Surgery

Robert M. Kershner, MD, FACS

General Considerations

Lens extraction with implantation of an intraocular lens is the most commonly performed refractive procedure in the world today. Since the invention of the intraocular lens in 1949 by the late Mr. Harold Ridley of England, lens implantation has become the primary procedure for the most common surgically corrected refractive error, aphakia, which occurs as a result of cataract extraction. I have published my experiences and clinical results on the technique of clear corneal cataract surgery correcting myopia, hyperopia and astigmatism since 1994. The results then, as today, demonstrate that we do a good job of improving people's visual acuity with the cataract procedure. It has only gotten better. Cataract surgery more often is considered a refractive procedure that optimizes uncorrected visual acuity, than solely as a surgical treatment for blindness due to a clouded crystalline lens.

Refractive Error Correction

LASIK has gained in popularity over the past decade. Along with myopia and hyperopia, astigmatism is one of the common indications for use of this procedure. Lasik is not the only approach to this problem, of course. It is however, one of the most expensive, requiring specialized equipment, skills, and includes the additional risks of creating a corneal flap and of removing corneal tissue without compromising corneal integrity. Surgeons who are proficient at handling the cornea during surgical procedures can embrace an additional approach to the correction of refractive errors. Today's advanced cataract procedure with high technology ("premium") IOL implantation, can fill the need. Corrective refractive surgery with implantable lenses has advanced substantially in this era of the correction of presbyopia, the natural loss of accommodative ability that comes with age.

Incisional Astigmatism Correction

Small incision surgery has motivated the IOL industry to develop newer acrylic, thermoplastic and liquid hydrogel materials that can correct spherical and astigmatic error through the smallest of microincisions. Coincident with these advances in microincision cataract surgery has been the increasingly superior visual results that patients have achieved. Myopia and hyperopia are eliminated with the IOL and astigmatism can be corrected with arcuate keratotomy incisions (the so-called limbal or peripheral corneal relaxing incisions – **Figure 1)**, the use of a toric IOL at the time of surgery, or excimer laser pre or postoperatively. Smaller incision surgery has meant better results for patients and less complications and worry for the surgeon.

Patients can expect to be spectacle-free for most tasks and read without the need for additional spectacle correction. The refractive outcome achieved with these techniques are the best we have ever achieved, and with incision sizes approaching one millimeter, this technology holds promise for even greater advances in the not too distant future **(Figures 2 – 4)**.

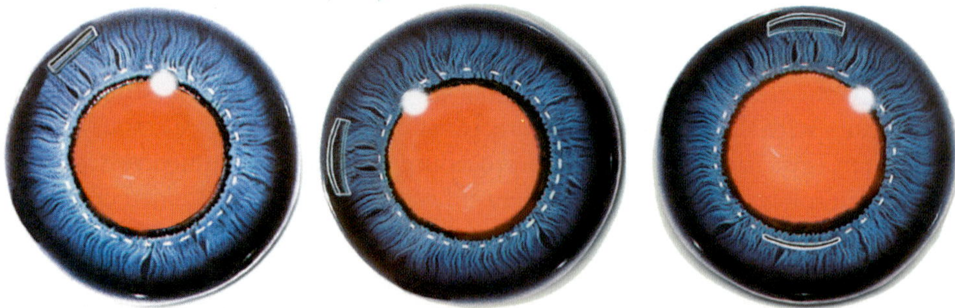

Figure 1: Location and architecture of clear corneal arcuate astigmatic incisions. Kershner. a) Single, clear corneal 2.5 mm planar, stab incision on the oblique or temporal limbus for astigmatic neutrality. b) Single, clear corneal 2.5 mm arcuate incision on the steepest axis at the 10mm optical zone to correct 1 D or less of astigmatism or a single 3.0 mm arcuate incision on the steepest axis at a 9 mm optical zone, to correct 1-2 D of astigmatism. c) Two arcuate keratotomy incisions are placed according to the nomograms to correct greater than 2 D of astigmatism. (Reprinted from: Kershner, RM. "Clear Cornea Cataract Surgery and the Correction of Myopia, Hyperopia and Astigmatism." Ophthalmology 1997;104:381-389.)

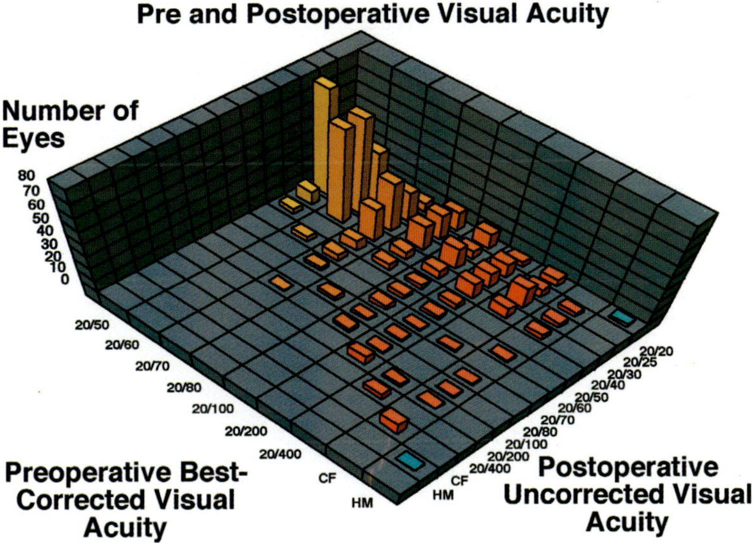

Figure 2: Comparison of preoperative best corrected and postoperative uncorrected visual acuity. n=690. Kershner. (Reprinted from: Kershner, RM. "Clear Cornea Cataract Surgery and the Correction of Myopia, Hyperopia and Astigmatism." Ophthalmology 1997;104:381-389.)

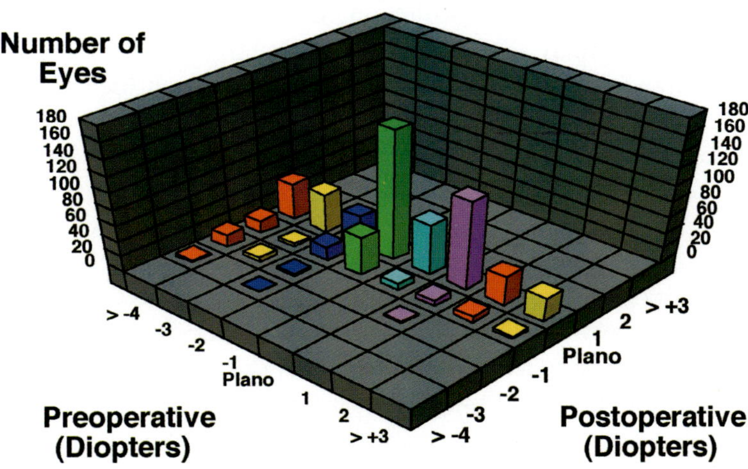

Figure 3: Comparison of preoperative and postoperative refractive sphere (D). Kershner. (Reprinted from: Kershner, RM. "Clear Cornea Cataract Surgery and the Correction of Myopia, Hyperopia and Astigmatism." Ophthalmology 1997;104: 381-389.)

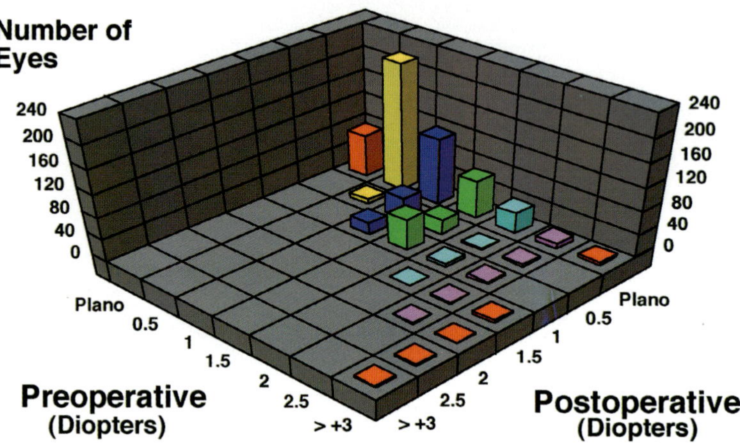

Figure 4: Comparison of preoperative and postoperative refractive cylinder (D). Kershner. (Reprinted from: Kershner, RM. "Clear Cornea Cataract Surgery and the Correction of Myopia, Hyperopia and Astigmatism." Ophthalmology 1997;104:381-389.)

Preoperative Evaluation and Surgical Plan

All patients who present for cataract surgery should undergo a comprehensive ophthalmic evaluation which includes dilated funduscopy. This seems self-evident, but sadly should never be assumed. I cannot begin to stress enough the importance of evaluating the entire patient, which includes each segment of the eye, that participates in refractive correction. All too often, I am called upon as an expert in the defense of a surgeon, who has either neglected to identify a pre-existing ocular disease, (corneal, retinal, or ocular pressure), or failed to follow-up on a finding discovered prior to surgery. In devising the surgical plan, cycloplegic refraction, combined with corneal topography and wavefront analysis, and ultrasonic biometry, is used to determine the best refractive approach and the best IOL power for complete refractive correction. The more data going into the surgery, the more likely that satisfactory correction will result. Few surgeons plan to fail, but many surgeons fail to plan. Know what it is exactly that you are setting out to correct and then aim for that outcome. If the goal of astigmatic treatment is to fully correct or slightly under-correct the cylinder, then make sure that the procedure doesn't overcorrect the power or shift the cylinder axis. To achieve the proper correction, a preoperative surgical plan must be developed and employed (See worksheets, **Table 1)**.

Table 1

Kershner Operative Worksheet

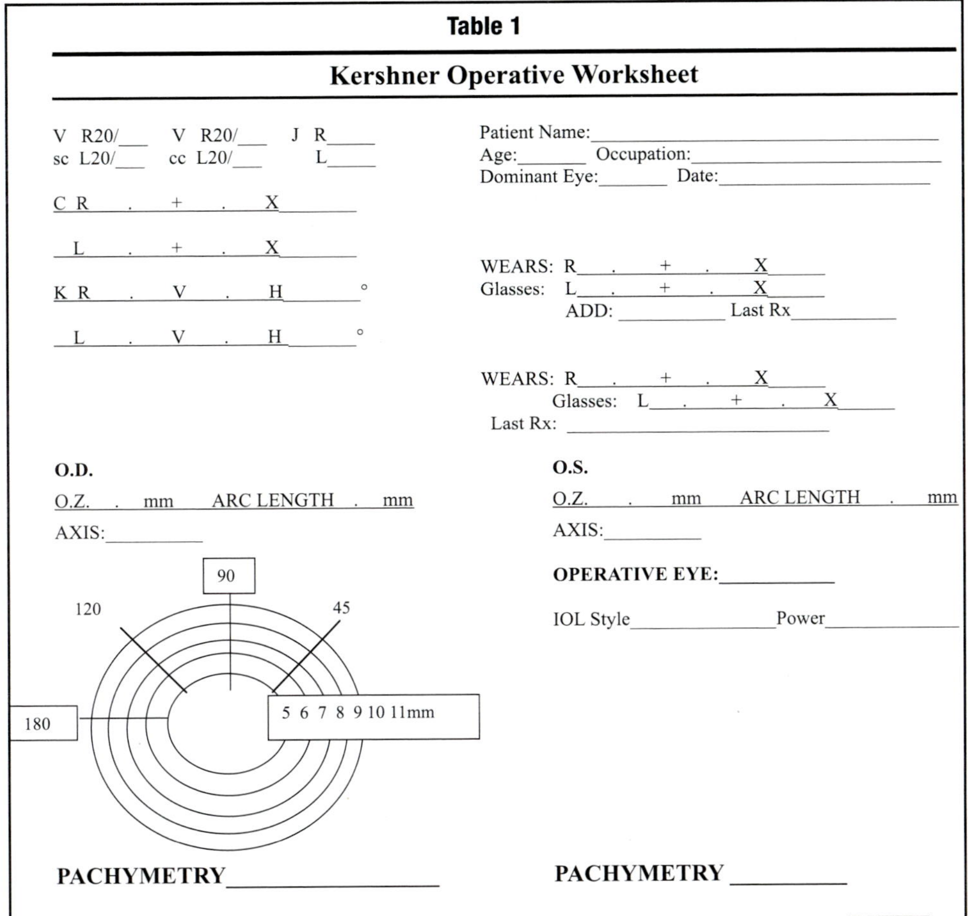

The Procedure

Use Topical Anesthesia

Topical anesthesia is quick, easy and effective. Patients trust the surgeon. If you use eyedrops to numb the eye, make sure to inform the patient that although they will feel pressure, see the light of the operating microscope, and feel the surgeon touching them, they will not have pain. If they think they won't feel anything, then they will startle the first time you touch the eye or eyelids, and they will no longer trust you. I always tell the patient when I am about to insert the specula, and start the phacoemulsification procedure, as insertion of the tip and the beginning of infusion causes a proprioceptive sensation of pressure. I inform them when I am about to inject the IOL, as the bag distends, they feel that stretch pressure as well. As long as the patient is informed, they will be content with what you have done. After all, they want you to succeed and they will always tolerate a little discomfort if they know to expect it and it will be worth it in the end.

After cycloplegia is instilled (and I prefer very short acting cycloplegia, such as tropicamide) and surgical scrub is completed, I instill several drops of 2.5% proparacaine or tetracaine HCL. Avoid the longer acting anesthetics such as bupivacaine as they are hyperosmotic, and will burn upon instillation and last longer than is necessary. My assistant applies a single drop of sterile 2.5% hydroxyl-propylmethylcellulose, (HPMC). Coating the cornea with HPMC rather than directing a stream of balanced salt solution over the ocular surface, avoids corneal epithelial disruption and patient discomfort. It also provides the added benefit of 1.5X magnification and improved visualization through the microscope.

Pay Attention to Your Incision-Use SLICK

Unlike scleral tunnel incisions, corneal incisions are not very forgiving. Operating on the primary refractive surface of the eye, it's easy to distort, tear, or stretch a corneal incision, and when you do, it will leak, induce unwanted astigmatism, and heal more slowly. The important features of incision construction are what I call the SLICK incision-Size, Location, Incision Configuration, and Keratotomy. Here are a few basic rules:

Size. A common error when constructing clear corneal incisions is to use a keratome that's too small for the instruments that will pass through the incision. This causes stretching or tearing and corneal striae that can obscure visualization during the procedure. It can also cause post-operative refractive and healing problems. Unlike scleral incisions, corneal incisions do not snap back into place after stretching. If your incision is too small, it will gape like a fish mouth rather than seal shut like a paper cut. The easiest way to avoid this is to use a keratome that is properly sized to accommodate your largest instrument **(Figure 5)**. Typically, corneal incisions wider than 3.2 mm will induce flattening and unwanted aberration in the refractive power of the central cornea. These incisions usually do not seal on their own, and may require suturing. Incisions 2.5 mm wide or less, seal appropriately and can be used to control the corneal curvature.

Location. Just as in real estate, location, location, location-where you place the incision is every bit as important as how you make it.

Incision Configuration. Only very sharp keratomes atraumatically penetrate Descemet's membrane. Many clear cornea surgeons use diamond blades because of their unrivaled sharpness. The cutting edges can be as thin as 1 μm, enabling these knives to pass through the corneal lamella smoothly and easily, leaving behind an incision that is undisrupted.

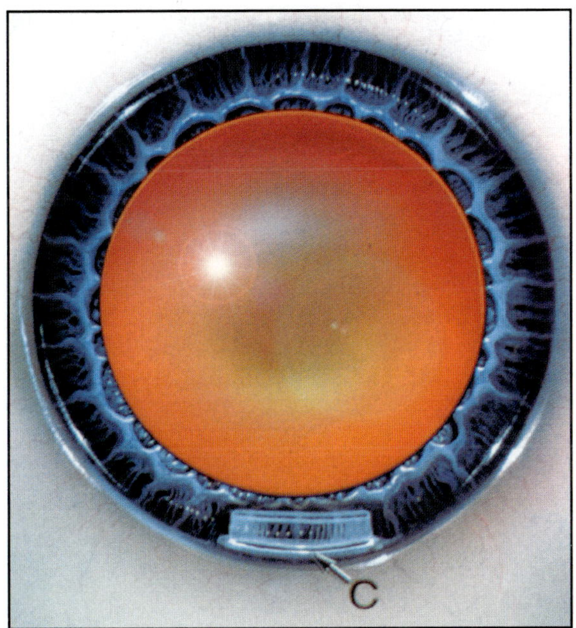

Figure 5: Corneal Tunnel Sutureless Incision. The 3.2 mm corneal tunnel incision (C) creates a valve which is self-sealing. If a corneal incision is made and the surgeon has to convert, the enlargement of the corneal incision to finish the operation as an extracapsular may lead to major astigmatism. It is preferible to close it and create a new superior scleral incision. (Art from Jaypee-Highlights Medical Publishers).

To assure proper geometry and architecture, place the tip of the corneatome on the incision entrance line, aim and line up the blade with the second line mark, then pass the blade into the cornea until it reaches the laser mark on the blade. At this point, the tip will enter the eye at the proper angle and the ideal tunnel length will be achieved automatically. The width to length ratio will be maintained at 3:2, which has been proven to be stable **(Figure 6)**.

Keratomes are available in a variety of widths to accommodate whatever phacoemulsification tip and lens insertion method you use. The ideal knife has a specially designed double-bevel slit blade, either angled or straight, for proper clear cornea incision construction. An accurate depth blade preset to 550 or 600 microns is used to construct the first step of the two-step arcuate keratotomy incision **(Figure 7)**.

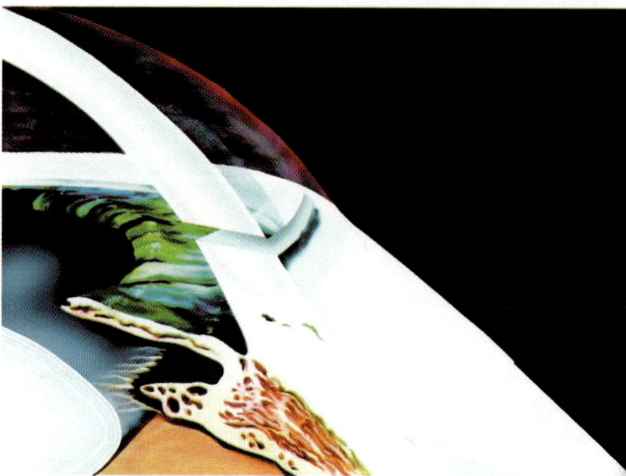

Figure 6: A single-plane incision is best for astigmatic neutrality. (Kershner)

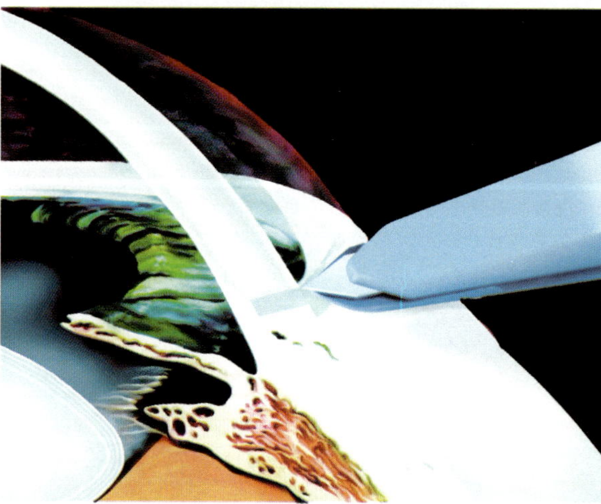

Figure 7: A two-step incision, with a vertical groove, maximizes achieved flattening. (Kershner)

Correct Astigmatism-Fix it, Don't Make it Worse

Where you place the incision is just as important as how you make it. Prior to surgery note in the chart the position of the patient's steepest meridian on the cornea (see worksheet- **Table 1)**. As all transverse or arcuate corneal incisions flatten the dome of the cornea, locate your incision on the steepest meridian. Can't determine where the steepest meridian is located? Simply refract the patient in plus cylinder or refer to a corneal topographic map. Remember this: Placing the incision anywhere other than the steepest meridian of the cornea will always make the astigmatism worse. Since most elderly patients have against-the-rule astigmatism, temporal incisions typically work best for most, but not all patients. These incisions are also a good choice if the patient has a spherical cornea. The temporal limbus, located further away from the optical center than the superior limbus, will induce less corneal astigmatism when incised. Patients with significant pre-existing astigmatism will benefit from astigmatic keratotomy at the time of surgery **(Table 2)**.

Table 2
Keratolenticuloplasty Procedure

1. The goal of surgery is to undercorrect the pre-existing astigmatism. You can always do more surgery later if needed, but it may be difficult to undo what you have already done if you have done too much and overcorrected the cylinder or shifted the axis. Remember, in older patients, the less elastic cornea responds with greater changes in curvature for a given amount of surgery.

2. Keep the incisions at the limbus or slightly onto the dome of the cornea. Avoid arcuate incisions inside the 7-mm optical zone. If it is possible to achieve the same degree of correction with a larger arc at a 10mm optical zone at the limbus, this is to be preferred over a smaller arc at a 8-mm or 9-mm optical zone. Larger incisions are always preferred further away from the optical zone than smaller arcs nearer the central cornea. Remember, the effect of corneal incisions to flatten decreases as the distance from the optical zone increases.

3. Arcuate incisions should never exceed 600 in length at any optical zone and, ideally, the largest arc should be no greater than 450 or 3.5 mm at an optical zone of 10mm.

4. To achieve the maximum flattening and best neutralize the astigmatism, incise the cornea to a depth of 85% to 95% of corneal thickness. Measure pachymetry at the proposed incision site and set the diamond blade to 90% of this measurement or simply use the disposable accurate depth metal blade preset at 550 or 600 microns. Do not over cut into cornea as perforating the cornea makes phacoemulsification and maintaining the anterior chamber more difficult. If perforation should occur, it may be necessary to suture the incision. This will diminish corneal flattening, but the suture can be removed at the slitlamp in a few days.

5. Whenever possible, a single arcuate incision will be preferable to using two smaller incisions.

6. Always use the arcuate incision closest to the surgeon for the keratotomy into the anterior chamber. Place this incision anterior to the limbal vascular arcade at a 11mm, 10 mm, or 9 mm optical zone. Avoid using the arcuate incision for the subsequent cataract surgery if it is closer to the optical center of the eye than the 8-mm optical zone.

7. To avoid full thickness penetration, avoid pressing on the globe with another instrument during the creation of the arcuate incision. To stabilize the eye use the disposable fixation ring if needed. Mark the proposed position of the incision at the steepest plus-cylinder reading.

8. It is easier to visualize the marks and incise the cornea if the cornea is kept dry. Avoid using marking inks. They obscure visualization for subsequent procedures of cataract surgery. A clean marker gently pressed onto the epithelium will create a visible mark that will be more than satisfactory as a guideline to creating the incision.

9. Always place the arcuate corneal cataract incision on the axis of steepest (+) astigmatism. Operating on the incorrect axis will always make the refractive result worse. Axis is crucial. Never operate greater than 15° off axis.

10. Keep the keratome fully applanated perpendicular to the surface of the cornea. Aim the blade towards the center of the globe and follow the curvature of the cornea closely following the mark until the full excursion of the incision is completed.

11. The slit blade, sized for the phacoemulsification tip and injection system, is placed at the base of the arcuate incision to enter the eye plane-parallel to the iris. The handle should be aimed at the center of the pupil to assure an incision which self-seals and has the proper architecture for the best refractive result.

How do arcuate astigmatism incisions differ from limbal relaxing incisions? Limbal relaxing incisions, because they are placed in the far periphery of the cornea at the scleral limbus, have less flattening effect for a given length. As a result, they must be large enough in length to have any substantial effect on corneal curvature. When limbal incisions traverse 120 degrees or arc, they have the significant downside of effectively denervating the cornea. In an elderly patient, this can result in an anesthetic cornea, severe dry eye, and corneal breakdown. Smaller, arcuate incisions have more effect with less surgery, and as long as they do not approach the optical center of the cornea, are much less problematic to create, and work through **(Tables 3A and 3B)**.

Table 3A

Kershner Arcuate Keratotomy Incision-Only System Nomograms			
Correction (Diopters)	Optical Zone (mm)	Number of Incisions	Arcuate Incision Length (mm)
<1.0	10	1	2.5
1.0	9	1	2.5
1.5	9	1	3,0
2.0	8	2	2.5
2.5	8	2	3.0
3.0	7	2	2.5
3.5	7	2	3.0
4,0	6 10	1 1	2,5 2.5
4.5	6 10	1 1	3.0 2.5
5.0	6 10	1 1	3.0 2.5
5.5	5 10	1 1	2.5 2.5
6.0	5 10	1 1	3.0 3.0

This nomogram is to be used when incisions alone are utilized to correct the cylinder. They are a guideline only, surgeons should adjust for the desired result. Corrected for age 60 +. Arcs placed on steepest axis of astigmatism (plus cylinder). Pachymetry at incision site, keratome set to 95% of pachymetry (550-600 microns). Mark arcuate incisions and optical zone with Kershner One-Step Marker. Cataract keratotomy at 10 mm, 9 mm, or 8 mm only.

Table 3B

Kershner Arcuate Keratotomy
With Toric IOL System Nomograms

Correction (Diopters)	Optical Zone (mm)	Number of Incisions	Arcuate Incision Length(mm)	Toric IOL
<1.0	10	1	2.5	
1.0	9	1	2.5	
1.5	9	1	3.0	+2.00 Toric
2.0	9	1	3.0	+2.00 Toric
2.5	9	1	3.0	+3.50 Toric
3.0	9	2	3.5	+3.50 Toric
3.5	8	1	3.0	+3.50 Toric
	10	1	3.0	
4.0	8	1	3.5	
	10	1	3.5	
4.5	8	1	4.0	
	10	I	4.0	
5.0	8	1	4.5	
	10	1	4,5	
5.5	8	1	5.0	
	10	1	5.0	
6.0	8	1	5.5	
	10	1	5.5	

This nomogram is to he used when incisions are utilized in combination with the toric IOL to correct the cylinder, They are to be used as a guideline only, surgeons should adjust for the desired result. Corrected for age 60. Arcs placed on steepest axis of astigmatism (plus cylinder). Pachymetry at incision site, keratome set to 95% of pachymetry (550-600 microns). Mark arcuate incisions and optical zone with Kershner One-Step Marker. Cataract keratotomy at 10 mm, 9 mm, or 8 mm only.

The Strategy for Achieving the Best Refractive Outcome from the Clear Cornea Refractive Cataract Procedure

Surgeons slow to accept the techniques of astigmatism management with their cataract procedure due to reluctance to acquire new skills, or new instrumentation, are depriving themselves and their patients of the potential for better refractive outcomes. Astigmatism should be managed, because it is better for our patients and is predictably and easily corrected with simple techniques. Adopt a few sound fundamental principles, use a paucity of additional instrumentation, and every surgeon can offer a better refractive result. The surgical correction of astigmatism along with full refractive correction of the sphere, reduces the need for spectacle correction postoperatively. Set your goal at achieving better refractive outcomes, and apply a philosophy of refractive correction with three simple rules:

Rule #1. Do not overcorrect the cylinder or shift it from it's pre-existing axis.

Rule #2. Accurately correct astigmatism, but first, accurately measure it.

Rule #3. Make the astigmatic correction on the proper meridian.

How do we Measure Astigmatism?

A full and accurate cycloplegic refraction allows us to determine the magnitude and the direction of the cylinder axis. Corneal topography and other corneal scanning methods can allow us to properly analyze the origin of the astigmatism. An individual who has a refractive cylinder that does not appear on topographic imaging (such as lenticular in origin) would not require an intervention on the cornea to correct it. Simply removing the cataract will suffice. If the topographic astigmatism, which is usually measured as less than the refractive astigmatism, does not correlate with the orientation of the refractive cylinder, then the surgeon must pass judgment on which refractive error to correct. Here is where the art of astigmatic correction with cataract surgery departs from it's science. The surgeon must be aware that using a cookbook approach for every patient will not work. It is always better to not attempt correction than perform the wrong treatment.

Topography can be valuable in both determining the qualitative appearance of the astigmatism as well as the location of the cylinder **(Figure 8)**, for selecting symmetrical or asymmetrical incisions. Newer methods of combined corneal and intraocular analysis (wavefront) provides insight into higher order aberrations that could also impact the postoperative refractive result. If the astigmatism is regular, it is correctable. Irregular astigmatism, keratoconus, corneal scars, and higher order aberrations are best left alone rather than to attempt a correction that could result in an undesirable postoperative irregular cornea.

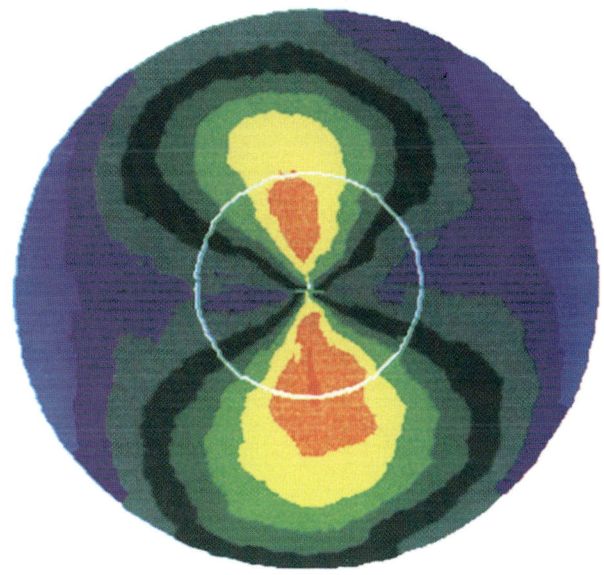

Figure 8: Preoperative topography shows an ideal candidate for refractive correction with cataract surgery. (Kershner)

How to Correct Astigmatism?

Early methods of astigmatic control at the time of surgery utilized suturing techniques and corneal wedge resection. Although this worked in instances where large corneal incisions were utilized for cataract surgery, it has no role in today's more precise techniques. The fundamental rule of "incisions placed onto the dome of the cornea will act as if tissue is added where they are placed". We can exploit this principle to flatten the steep areas of the cornea to create a more spherical one. Small, arcuate corneal incisions work best. Arcuate incisions, which closely follow the corneal curvature, placed on the proper latitude, flatten in the meridian in which they are placed. This neutralizes preexisting corneal astigmatism **(Table 3A-B)**. Flattening in one meridian results in a steepening of the meridian 90º away, a coupling ratio of approximately 1:1. One of the benefits of this principle is that the overall spherical error and the IOL power DO NOT CHANGE, as the net effect of correcting the astigmatism on sphere is zero.

We maximize the effect of the clear corneal cataract incision by inducing the flattening in the meridian in which it is placed. Simply by operating on the steepest meridian, improves the refractive results in most patients. Operate more than 15º off axis, however, and you will make always add to the astigmatism and the postoperative refractive result will be undesirable. That is why it is critical to know the location of the proper meridian on which to operate. In evaluating the patient for refractive cataract surgery, I take into account the cycloplegic refraction, topography, wavefront analysis and A-scan. The proper IOL is then selected based upon multiple measurements and the location of the steep astigmatic meridian is clearly marked on the chart in red. To take that information with you to identify the proper meridian in the operating room, surgeons should note in the chart any identifying characteristic that won't move when the patient is supine (see the worksheet in this chapter-Table 1) noting the presence of a small nevus or corkscrew vessel which may help identify the 12:00 o'clock meridian, for example. Using this as a guide, the proper meridian for the astigmatic correction can be selected. I prefer to use an ocular reticule in the operating microscope that allows me to align the proper axis with the microscope. Alternatively, the surgeon can use a hand-held degree gauge, or intraoperative keratometer to determine the proper meridian. Rotational movement of the eye when the patient is supine is not an issue when topical anesthesia is used. If a peribulbar or retrobulbar block is administered however, this potential error should be compensated for when determining the proper location for incisional correction. It is best to mark the axis prior to the administration of any injection anesthetic block.

Here is how we maximize the effect of the clear corneal incision to flatten the cornea with the incision:

For astigmatically neutral clear corneal incisions, a one-step plane-parallel clear corneal incision is fashioned (Figures 1 and 7). A 2.4 mm disposable keratome can be used to create the proper architecture for a clear corneal incision that will be self-sealing which maintains the magic ratio of 3:2, width to length. If the width of the incision is 3 mm, the tunnel length through the cornea should be approximately 2 mm. In keratolenticuloplasty, the cataract incision is used to optimize the refractive result. The cataract incision itself can correct up to 1.0 diopters (D) of astigmatism when created in a length of approximately 3mm or less (Figure 1). For an astigmatically neutral incision (A) a single-plane parallel incision is created with the keratome. For less than 1D of astigmatism, (B) a two-step clear corneal incision is utilized to flatten in the meridian in which it is placed. Use a calibrated, accurate depth blade, set at a depth of 550 to 600 microns, and make the incision vertical, perpendicular to the cornea. Position the blade handle towards the center of the globe to create a deep groove approximately 85% of corneal depth. Use a corneatome that meets the dimensions for the phaco tip and the IOL injector. Enter the eye plane parallel, creating a two-step clear corneal self-sealing incision is with the maximum flattening effect.

To correct larger degrees of astigmatism, (C) the incision is combined with an additional arcuate incision on the opposite meridian from the cataract incision, at an optical zone of 9, 10 or 11mm to induce further flattening, or it may be combined with the implantation of a toric intraocular lens.

Conclusions

Today's advanced surgical techniques of microincision cataract surgery have enabled surgeons to fully correct refractive error with cataract removal and the selective use of advanced optic technology and toric IOL implantation. Smaller, more flexible and injectable intraocular lenses, combined with more efficient methods of phacoemulsification have made it possible to keep incision sizes less than 2.0 mm, and as small as 1 mm. Judicious selection of the intraocular IOL and careful attention to astigmatic correction, maximizes the full refractive potential for each cataract patient. Patients should expect more with these techniques, as they benefit from highly accurate refractive corrections, unheard of just a few short years ago, less postoperative complications, less need for postoperative care, and less need for optical correction following surgery.

Editorial Comment

Nowadays, a satisfactory refractive result after a cataract surgery is as important as the absence of complications during its procedure. In this context there are two major factors to be taken into account: First, it is imperative to perform an excellent biometry in order to achieve a very accurate dioptric power calculation of the intraocular lens that is to be implanted, and second, the existing pre-surgical corneal astigmatism must be measured and corrected. An accurate pre-surgical (with and without) cycloplegic refraction, corneal keratometry, corneal topography, corneal and ocular wavefront aberrometry are important information needed to measure the magnitude of the astigmatism, its location, its symmetry, and to determine whether it is regular or irregular. All this information is employed in the planning of the treatment at the time of the cataract surgery, whether it is to be performed with the use of corneal incisions (either limbal relaxing incisions or arcuate astigmatic incisions), or with the use of a toric IOL, or with the use of both techniques.

Arnaldo Espaillat, MD

Bibliography

1. Kershner, RM. "Correction of Astigmatism with Clear-Corneal Cataract Surgery" Section IV. Managing Astigmatism in Cataract Surgery, In: Henderson, B, Gills J, eds. A Complete Surgical Guide for Correcting Astigmatism. Thorofare, NJ: Slack, Inc.; 2010: Chapter 8.
2. Kershner, RM. "Improved Functional Vision with a Modified Prolate IOL," "New Technology IOLs," "Ophthalmic Viscosurgical Devices: Seven Secrets to their Success,"and "HydroLasik," Bringing You the Future in Ophthalmology-2005, Pierre Faber and Michel Giunta, moderators, Mediconcept, Inc. Montreal, Quebec, Canada, 2005.

3. Kershner, RM. "Optimizing the Refractive Outcome: Correction of Astigmatism in Cataract Surgery" In The Highlights Collection - New Outcomes in Cataract Surgery, Highlights of Ophthalmology International (Panama) Chapter 2, pp. 15-28, 2005.

4. Kershner, RM. "Foreword" In Step by Step Phaco, Agarwal, Agarwal, and Agarwal. New Delhi, India: Jaypee Brothers, 2005.

5. Kershner, RM "Management of the Small Pupil in Clear Cornea Cataract Surgery" in Pandey, Suresh, A Surgeon's Guide to Phacoemulsification, Slack, Inc., 2004.

6. Kershner RM. Correction of astigmatism in clear cornea cataract surgery. In: Gills J, ed. A Complete Surgical Guide for Correcting Astigmatism. Thorofare, NJ: Slack, Inc.; 2002: Chapter 7, pp.49-64.

7. Kershner, RM "Management of the Small Pupil for Clear Corneal Cataract Surgery" Phaco, Phakonit and Laser Phaco-A Quest for the Best, Eds. Agarwal, S, Agarwal, A, Agarwal, A., Highlights of Ophthalmology International (Panama) Chapter 20, pp. 213-220, 2002.

8. Kershner, RM "Optimizing the Refractive Outcome of Clear Cornea Cataract Surgery" Phaco, Phakonit and Laser Phaco-A Quest for the Best, Eds. Agarwal, S, Agarwal, A, Agarwal, A., Highlights of Ophthalmology International (Panama), Chapter 9, pp. 85-104, 2002.

9. Kershner RM. "Single Instrument Phacoemulsification" Phacoemulsification, Laser Cataract Surgery and Foldable IOLs 2nd Edition, Eds. Agarwal, Agarwal, Sacedev, Fine and Agarwal. New Delhi, India: Jaypee Brothers, 2000, pp. 146-150.

10. Kershner RM. "Clear Corneal Incision System for Cataract Surgery" Refractive Surgery Eds Agarwal, Agarwal, Agarwal. New Delhi, India: Jaypee Brothers, 1999

11. Kershner RM. "Phacoemulsification Through a Clear Corneal Microincision" Phacoemulsification, Laser Cataract Surgery and Foldable IOLs Eds. Agarwal, Agarwal, Sacedev, Fine and Agarwal. New Delhi, India: Jaypee Brothers,1998, pp. 118-114

12. Kershner, RM. "Clear Corneal Refractive Cataract Surgery" Clinical and Surgical Ophthalmology 2006;24(2):46-54.

13. Kershner RM. "Refractive Clear Cornea Cataract Surgery." Ophthalmic Practice 2002; 20(7):1-5.

14. Kershner, RM. "Toric Lenses for Correcting Astigmatism in 130 Eyes." Discussion, Ophthalmology, 2000;107:1776-82.

15. Kershner, RM. "Six Tips to Clear Cornea Cataract Surgery." Review of Ophthalmology, VI(4):120-124, April, 1999.

16. Kershner, RM. "Refractive Cataract Surgery" in Current Opinion in Ophthalmology, Richard Lindstrom, ed. Pennsylvania: Thompson Science 9(1):46-54, February 1998.

17. Kershner, RM. "Patient's Adaptation to Cataract Surgery" Ophthalmology 1998;105(1):6-7.

18. Kershner, RM. "Clear Corneal Cataract Surgery and the Correction of Myopia, Hyperopia and Astigmatism." Ophthalmology 1997; 104(3):381-389.

19. Kershner RM. "Topical Anesthesia Cataract Surgery." Ophthalmic Practice 1993; 11(4):160-165.

20. Kershner RM. "Antibacterial Prophylaxis Before, During and After Routine Cataract Surgery." in Consultative Section, edited by Samuel Masket, M.D. Journal of Cataract and Refractive Surgery 1993; 19(1):110.

21. Kershner RM. "Capsular Rupture at Hydrodissection." Journal of Cataract and Refractive Surgery 1992; 18:201.

22. Kershner RM. "Topical Anesthesia for Small Incision Self-Sealing Cataract Surgery - A Prospective Study of the First 100 Patients." Journal of Cataract and Refractive Surgery 1993; 19(3):290-292.

23. Kershner, RM. "Sutureless one-handed intercapsular phacoemulsification: The keyhole technique." J Cataract Refract Surg 1991;17(suppl):719-25.

24. Kershner, RM. "Embryology, anatomy and needle capsulotomy." In: Koch PS, Davison JA, eds. Textbook of Advanced Phacoemulsification Techniques. Thorofare, NJ: Slack, 1991;35-48.

25. Kershner, RM. "Keratolenticuloplasty: Arcuate keratotomy for cataract surgery and astigmatism." J Cataract Refract Surg 1995;21:274-7.

26. Kershner, RM. ed. Refractive Keratotomy for Cataract Surgery and the Correction of Astigmatism. Thorofare, NJ: Slack, 1994.

3

IOL Power Calculation in Standard and Complex Cases

George O. Waring IV, MD

Introduction

Accurate biometry is the single most important factor in determining excellent outcomes with intraocular lens surgery. This is even more crucial with the advent of toric and presbyopia-correcting IOLs which are eliminating the distinction between refractive and cataract surgeons. Patient expectations are elevated when investing in premium technology. As no IOL is perfect, it is necessary to understand the patient's comprehension and tolerance for the trade-offs involved with any IOL and to establish realistic expectations. This is particularly true when patients have high degrees of refractive error, anomalous and post surgical eyes. Tracking patient outcomes can help identify the surgeon specific biometric patterns for each IOL. The purpose of this chapter is to educate cataract and lens surgeons on understanding the fundamentals and nuances of proper biometric evaluation, technique and decision making.

Evaluating the Patient Prior to Surgery

An initial and complete ocular evaluation should be performed, whereby the type and density of the cataract is determined with slit lamp biomicroscopy **(Figure 1A-D)**. Adjunctive tools such as Scheimpflug densitometry and double pass wavefronts can aid in assessment of a precataract or "dysfunctional lens" and

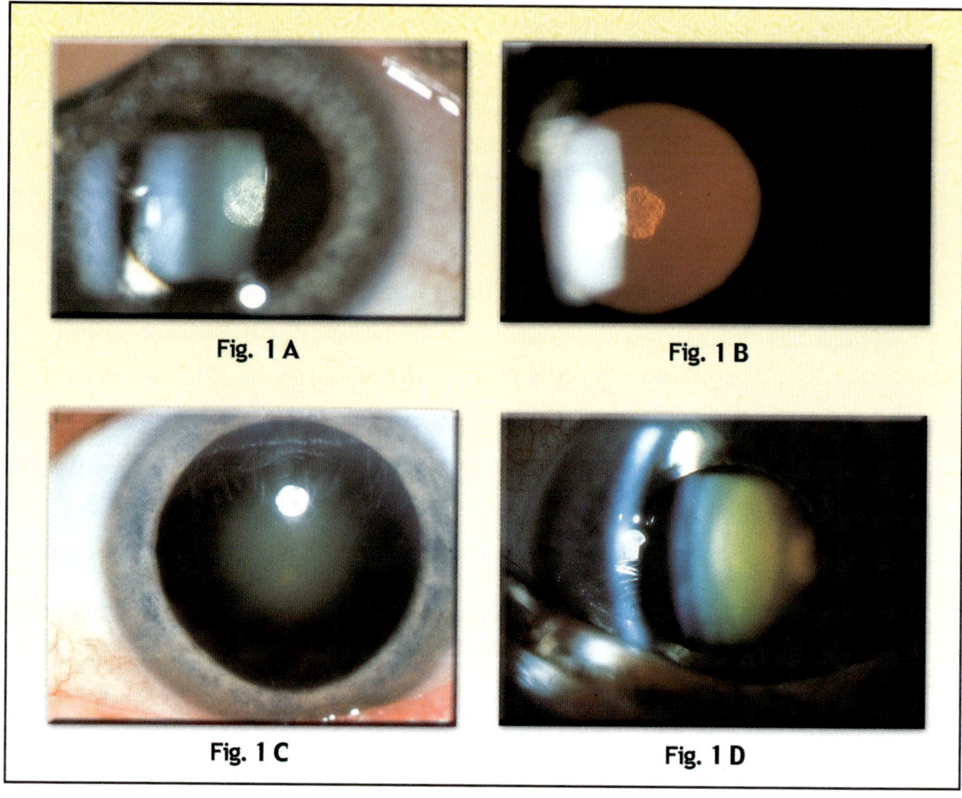

Figure 1 A-D: Posterior subcapsular cataract (top, left and right). Cataract with nuclear sclerosis (bottom, left and right). Figures 1A and B are three dimensional photographs of a characteristic posterior subcapsular cataract, seen with the slit lamp (top-left) and with indirect illumination also using the slit lamp (top-right). Figures 1C and D are three dimensional photos of nuclear sclerotic cataract, viewed with diffuse illumination (left) and with the slit lamp beam (right). This is the most common form of cataract. Patients tend to be hindered more by loss of contrast sensitivity rather than glare. (Reproduced with permission from AAO's Basic and Clinical Science Course, Lens and Cataract 2003, enhanced by Jaypee-Highlights).

can also augment the patient education process. A careful automated and manual calibrated keratometry is performed prior to taking the intraocular pressures, and a full dilated retinal exam should be done. A Potential Acuity Meter (PAM) can predetermine the expected outcome in the majority of surgical cases. Additional testing can include slit lamp digital photography, retinal digital photography, Optical Coherence Tomography (OCT), endothelial cell count, Optical or Contact Corneal Pachymetry (CCP). Topography and tomography are critical tools for premium IOLs and astigmatic correction.

Once the surgery is to be performed, the risks, complications and alternatives are explained. The expected postoperative refraction is determined. Careful discussion with the patient will help the surgeon understand the patient's expectations. Some patients know exactly what they want, while others will leave the decision up to their surgeon.

Patient's Expectations

It is essential to explore, discuss and define patient's expectations prior to surgery. Postoperative patient satisfaction is based on this pre-op surgeon-patient communication and understanding. The following questions should be considered: what are the patient's daily needs and what final uncorrected visual acuity for distance and near he would prefer? Do they want to read with less dependence on reading glasses? If so, they must understand they will not see clearly at distance, in the distance eye if they desire monovision. Myopic patients generally prefer to end up myopic. Hyperopes do better by performing eventual bilateral surgery. Low vision patients might prefer moderate myopic refractive outcome.

The availability of multifocal IOLs, accommodative implants, monovision, toric, and piggyback implantation have to be explained to the appropriate patients. Final visual satisfaction with these technologies will depend a great deal on the selection by the surgeon of the right patient with reasonable expectations, including but not limited to risk of dysphotopsias, limitations of refractive range, and possibility for lens exchange or surgical enhancement in the future

Typically, patients can tolerate a 1.5 to 2.0 D difference in refractive error between the two eyes (anisometropia), with minimal risks of asthenopia and / or diplopia. To achieve iseikonia, i.e., the equality of retinal image size, the two eyes should have equal posterior focal lengths. In emmetropic eyes undergoing cataract surgery, iseikonia is typically preserved when IOL calculations aims towards emmetropia or even slight myopia. In eyes with large refractive errors, the problem becomes more complicated and specific formulas are needed for proper calculations to minimize appreciable image size disparity. The majority of patients are unaffected by aniseikonia of up to 5%, which reflects a refractive error variation of about 2.5 D. The iseikonic IOL power calculations should be carefully considered with both high degrees of bilateral refractive error with plananed unilateral surgery, or severe anisometropia.

The expected postoperative refractive error should be discussed with the patient prior to surgery. IOL power selection in emmetropes is relatively straight forward. Young, active emmetropes want to remain so, while older, sedentary patients may enjoy slight myopia. I typically perform cataract surgery in the non-dominant eye first, to make the proper final adjustments for the second eye at the time of the surgery, though recent studies have suggested that simultaneous bilateral cataract surgery does not reduce the IOL power calculation accuracy in the second eye.

Determining IOL Power (Biometry)

Biometry includes two fundamental components: keratometry and axial length. However, in clinical practice, the term biometry refers to the latter and keratometry is generally considered to be a separate process.

The modern methods for biometry include Partial Coherence Interferometry (now known as Optical Coherence Biometry) and Advanced Contact and Immersion Ultrasonography.

Postop Refractive Errors No Longer Admissible

This is particularly true considering increased patient's expectations and the minimal astigmatism created by small incision cataract surgery. It has been estimated that 70% of cataract patients have less than 1 diopter of preoperative astigmatism. Of the remaining patients, an estimated 20% have between 1 and 2 diopters, and may require additional astigmatism surgery such as Limbal Relaxing Incisions (LRIs), practiced today by about half of surgeons in the USA. The remaining 10% of patients have astigmatism higher than 2 diopters, and LRIs in these cases can become unpredictable. In these cases, toric IOL implantation or a bioptic procedure may produce the desired result.

Therefore, exact determination of the IOL power to match the specific planned postoperative refraction is the goal. The implantation of multifocal and accommodative IOLs, as well as performing surgery on eyes with different axial lengths: normal **(Figure 2)**, hyperopic **(Figure 3A-B)**, myopic **(Figure 4)** eyes, make these measurements even more important.

Partial Coherence Interferometry, now known as Optical Coherence Biometry (IOL Master) is quickly becoming the standard of care. Light has a shorter wavelength than ultrasound, allowing for a much higher axial resolution. It also has another major advantage in that it measures the "optical" axial length (corneal vertex to fovea) rather than the "anatomic" axial length measured by the ultrasound (corneal vertex to posterior pole). However, light is subject to bending when entering materials with different indices of refraction and ultrasound is more sensitive to detecting different optical surface interfaces. IOL Masters cannot be performed in 17% of eyes due to significant posterior subcapsular, dense cataracts or poor fixation.

The Challenge of Complex Cases

Corneal refractive surgery, including excimer refractive surgery **(Figure 6)**, radial keratotomy **(Figure 7)**, conductive keratoplasty, intracorneal ring segments **(Figure 8)** and inlays can make IOL power calculation more difficult with the uncertainty of the true corneal power and original corneal power. In these particular cases, tomography, topography and high resolution corneal OCT are indispensable for estimation of true corneal power.

IOL power calculation in pediatric cataract patients **(Figure 10)**, in eyes with previous vitreoretinal surgery and use of silicone oil **(Figure 11)**, in very short eyes **(Figures 3 A and B)**, in extremely long eyes **(Figure 4)**, in previous corneal transplant patients, secondary implantations, IOL exchange, previous vitrectomy, or when planning multifocal IOL implantation are some of the cases still considered to be challenging for calculations.

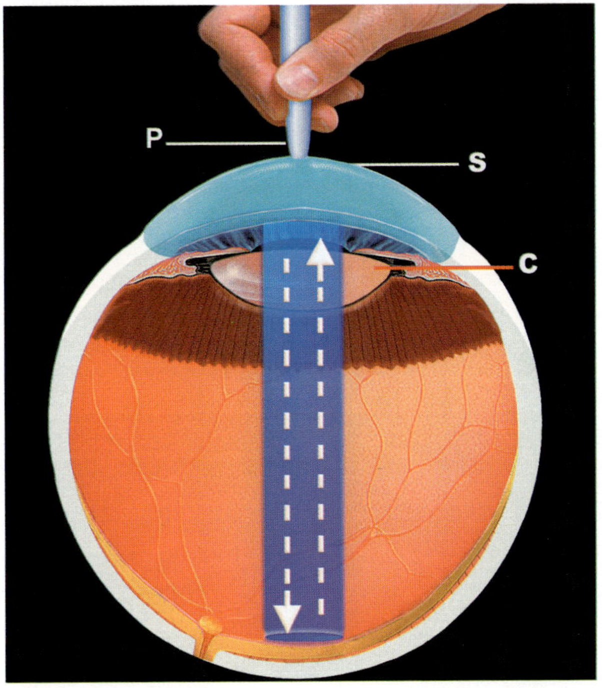

Figure 2: Determination of IOL power in patients with normal axial length (normal eyes) - Mechanism of how ultrasound measures distances and determines axial length. The use of ultrasound to calculate the intraocular lens power takes into account the variants that may occur in the axial length of the eye and the curvature of the cornea. The ultrasound probe (P) emits and receives high frequency sound waves. The sound waves travel through the eye until they are reflected back by any structure that stands perpendicularly in their way (represented by arrows). The speed of the ultrasound waves (arrows) is higher through a dense lens (C) than through a clear lens. Soft tipped transductors (P) are recommended to avoid errors when touching the corneal surface (S). The computer of the ultrasound unit can automatically multiply the time by the sound velocity to obtain the axial length. (Art from Jaypee-Highlights Medical Publishers, Inc.)

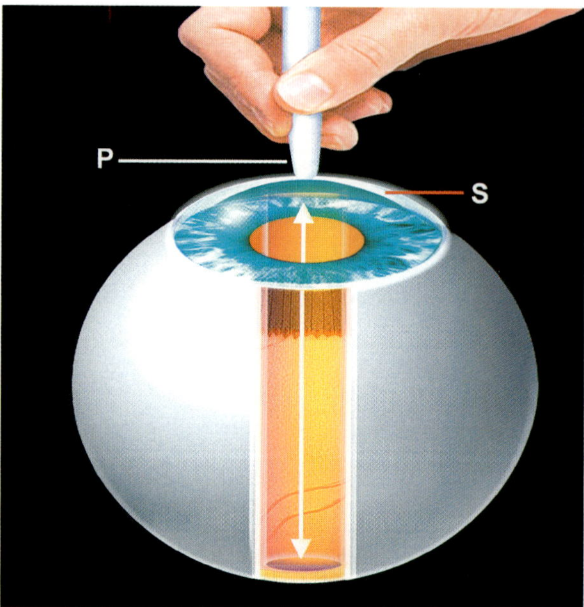

Figure 3A: IOL power calculation in patients with very short axial length (hyperopia). In eyes with short axial lengths, the third generation formulas such as the Holladay 2 and Hoffer-Q seem to provide the best results. Holladay found that the size of the anterior and posterior segments is not necessarily proportional in extremely short eyes (<20.0 mm). Only 20% of short eyes present a small anterior segment (nanophthalmic eyes); as 80% present a normal anterior segment and an abnormally short posterior segment as shown here. (P) represents probe, (S) represents corneal surface.   (Art from Jaypee-Highlights Medical Publishers, Inc.)

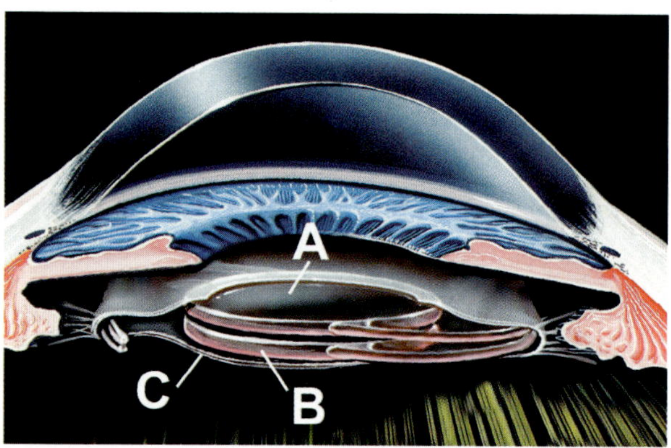

Figure 3B: Concept of the piggyback high plus intraocular lenses. In cases of very high hyperopia, lens extraction can be combined with piggyback intraocular lens implantation. One (A) or two (B) intraocular lenses can be implanted inside the capsular bag (C). We recommend implanting the first IOL in the bag and the second, anterior IOL in the sulcus to reduce the risk of interlenticular opacification. This piggyback implantation technique may solve the problems of having to implant a lens of over +40.0 diopters with its consequent optical aberrations. (Art from Jaypee-Highlights Medical Publishers, Inc.)

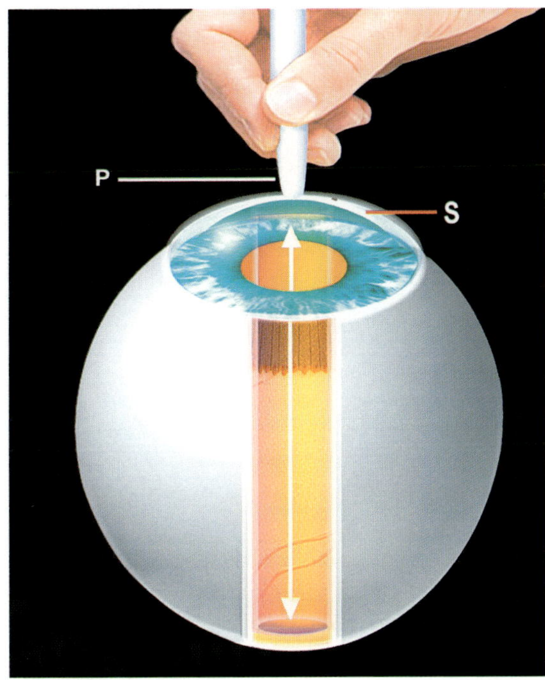

Figure 4: IOL power calculation in high myopia with axial lengths higher than 27.0mm the use of the SRK/T formula has shown good predictability. Probe (P), corneal surface (S). (Art from Jaypee-Highlights Medical Publishers, Inc.)

Axial length (AL) shoud be measured with the IOL Master (Partial Coherence Interferometry) when possible and/or immersion with ultrasonography as indicated. Bilateral measurements should be taken for comparison. If a disparity is found, this should be confirmed and correlated with refractive error, keratometry and visual acuity to account for the difference.

When using ultrasound, the axial length is determined by measurements obtained from the eye tissue interfaces with the ultrasound beam **(Figure 2 – arrows)**. The A- scan must be carefully calibrated and the velocity must correspond to whether or not the patient is phakic, pseudophakic, or aphakic and may need to be modified in some of the special cases previously described. When using an A-Scan Biometer there are components that the user must understand as the probe configuration, the transducer, the emitted ultrasound beam, the oscilloscope, the sensitivity setting, the velocity setting, the electronic gates, and the biometer's report **(Figure 5)**. Furthermore, the quality of waveforms should be critically evaluated on all scans. Sharp, well defined, tall peaks are desired and short or tall flat tops are not acceptable and should be repeated.

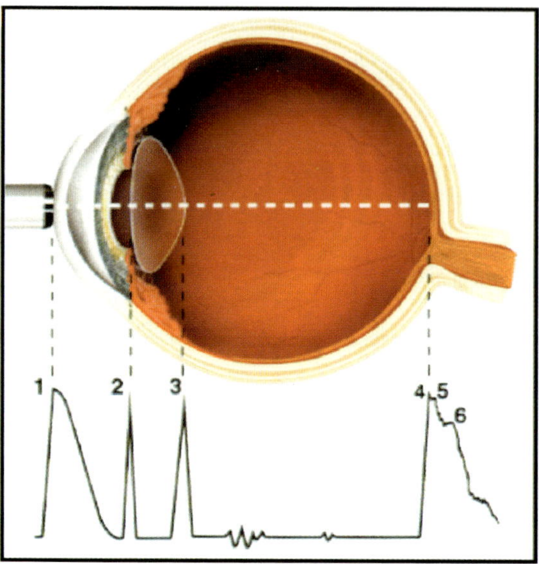

Figure 5: A Scan of a normal eye. 1. Cornea; 2. Anterior lens capsule; 3. Posterior lens capsule; 4. Retina; 5. Sclera; and 6. Orbital fat.

Most Commonly Used Formulas

There are two basic groups of formulas, the Theoretical and the Empirics (Regression) Formulas. At the present time, the most precise formulas are considered to be the Third Generation of the Theoretical Formulas and their variations, also known as Fourth Generation Theoretical Formulas. The Theoretical Formulas are based on geometrical optics. The various theoretical formulas differ in how they calculate the Estimated Lens Position (ELP), i.e. the IOL position related to the cornea. Accounting for ELP, is a key factor in determining accurate calculations. In the First Generation Theoretical formulas, the ELP (then ACD) was a constant factor depending of the IOL position (Fyodorov, Colenbrander, Hoffer, Thijssen, Van Der Heijde, and Binkhorst). The Second Generation related the ELP to the AL (Binkhorst, Shammas, and Hoffer). In the Third Generation, the ELP is based on function of the AL and Keratometry (Holladay I in 1988, SRK/T in 1990, Hoffer Q in 1993). The Fourth Generation Theoretic Formulas are based on the ELP calculation in more than two variables (Olsen in 1990, Holladay II in 1996). The Holladay II formula is included in the Holladay IOL Consultant software.

The Regression or Empiric Formulas are based on the retrospective statistical analysis of refractive results of multiple surgical procedures. In 1980, Sanders, Retzlaff and Kraff described the SRK formula, currently the commonly used formula: P = A-2.5 AL − 0.9 K. The constant A varies with the implant design, material and the manufacturer. Based on this formula, one should immediately appreciate the weighted importance of accurate axial length calculations in IOL power determination relative to keratometry, as a 1mm error in AL can result in approximately 2.5D IOL power error.

Within the normal range of axial length (22.0 to 24.5 mm), most formulas yield similar results, however the results will differ at the AL extremes. The SRK formula has been found to be reasonably accurate for eyes with axial lengths between 22mm and 24.5mm. These eyes constitute approximately 75% of cases, while 14% of cases have axial lengths greater than 24.5 mm, and 10% have axial lengths less than 22mm. In 1993 Hoffer published data on formula relative to axial lengths. In general, recommended formulas based on AL are presented below **(Table 1)**.

Table 1

Axial Length	< 22.0	22.0 – 24.0	> 24.0
Suggested Formula	Holladay II Modified Hoffer Q Haigis	Average Holladay I	SRK/T Holladay I

The "average" formula is obtained calculating the mean of the three formulas: Hoffer, Holladay and SRK/T.

Modified formulas were developed to correct for errors in these formulas occurring in long and short eyes. The SRK II formula is a modification of the original SRK formula with the addition of a correction factor that increases the lens power in short eyes and decreases it in long eyes. The suggested method of modification of SRK to SRK II is shown below **(Table 2)**.

Table 2

L (mm)	Add to 'A' constant
Less than 20.00	+ 3
20.00 - 20.99	+ 2
21.00 - 21.99	+ 1
Greater than 24.50	-0.5

Over the last few years, the Regression Formulas have been considered less predictable than the latest generation of Theoretic Formulas. The Hoffer Q, Holladay I and SRK/T are available in the Hoffer 2.5 software.

Primary Sources of Error

The most common source of postoperative refractive error is due to imprecise preoperative biometric measurements. From these causal errors in IOL power calculations, 68% are due to errors in axial length (AL) measurement, 22% are due to not using the appropriate formula, and 10% are attributed to incorrect keratometric readings (Olsen).

AL measurements have improved with increasing use of immersion and Partial Coherence Interferometry (IOL Master) technologies to the point where 85 to 90% cases will be within 1 diopter of the desired postoperative refraction.

Surgeons have access to advanced theoretical formulas with the incorporation of the Haigis formula within the IOL Master. The Holladay Consultant software contains the Holladay II formula and the recently released Hoffer 2.5 software, which utilizes the latest versions of the Average Formula, Hoffer Q, Holladay I, and SRK/T, **(Table 1)**.

Finally, keratometry should be critically evaluated. It is good practice to obtain manual and topographic / tomographic K's. Topography or tomography, should be evaluated for quality of maps, irregularities due to dry eye, anterior basement membrane dystrophy (ABMD), scars, or otherwise irregular or highly aberrated corneas. Scans should be taken after instillation of preservative free artificial tears in a dark environment as keratometry can vary significantly with dry eye. The ocular surface should be optimized with dry eye patients if irregularities are found on topography. Clinically significant ABMD should be treated with superficial keratectomy and allowed to stabilize prior to keratometry determination. Serial scans are a good idea with irregular corneas.

Targeting Post-Op Refraction

This parameter is determined by the treating physician and is programmed into the software for the IOL power calculation. All the other parameters, except the ELP, are measured or assumed values.

For distance correction or multifocal IOLs, I generally recommend a target of plano to -0.25, particularly in a previous emmetropic or hyperopic patient. For monovision (I prefer the term "blended vision") I generally target -1.25D, depending on the age and needs of the patient. It is worth mentioning that classically, the non-dominant eye is targeted for myopia in monovision, though a small portion of patients who are "near dominant" may prefer to have the dominant eye targeted for near. Dominance can be assessed through motor and optical blur testing methods, and optical should take precedence in the instance of disagreement between the two modalities. In myopic patients, we bias toward a slight myopic target, which depends on the individuals' goals and needs. Small amounts of myopic against the rule astigmatism may aid in near vision.

Patients with poor best corrected visual potential may benefit from a postoperative myopic target. It has been suggested that a 20/200 or 20/400 visual acuity potential, verified by PAM and clinical findings, can benefit from a -4.0 to -5.0 D of postoperative refraction.

Finally, patients should be counseled regarding the need of reading glasses or bifocals if they elect for plano target bilaterally with monofocal implants. Candidates for multifocal IOL implantation, accommodative IOL implantation or monovision, need extra chair time to thoroughly explain the benefits and potential side effects to these patients. If realistic expectations are not present, the surgeon should suggest another alternative instead of facing an eventually dissatisfied patient.

Monocular Correction

When assessing IOL power calculation in monocular patients, dense amblyopia, or limited visual acuity in one eye, a postoperative refraction of plano to -1.0 D is a reasonable choice. These patients should wear safety glasses, where one only correct for distance vision.

Binocular Correction

Good Vision in the Non-Operated Eye

When choosing IOL powers for planned monovision, the surgeon should aim for less than 2.0 D of difference between the two eyes. Greater than 2.0 D difference increases the risk of diplopia. Greater than a 2.5 D difference increases the risk of aniseikonia, resulting in asthenopia or rapid fatigue of the eyes accompanied with headaches. Remember to account for iseikonia with high refractive error with only one eye needing surgery.

These calculations are unnecesary if the refractive error in the fellow eye is corrected with a contact lens, corneal refractive surgery, or lens surgery in the fellow eye. To avoid anisometropia, in a patient who has good vision in the non-operative eye, one must then target the intraocular lens power for a refraction within two diopters of his/her present prescription in the non-operative eye. For example, in a patient with a unilateral cataract who wishes to only have surgery in his cataractous eye, and a manifest refraction of +5.0D of hyperopia OU, we should target the postoperative refraction in the eye with the cataract for +3.00D, so there is a 90% probability that there will be less than a 3 diopter difference. Otherwise the Hoffer's iseikonic formula or the Shammas iseikonic equations are utilized. Bilateral lens surgery with a plano target is an excellent option as well, and should be carefully considered in these cases.

In contrast, if the patient were highly myopic in each eye, for example, -10.00D in both eyes, we should target the intraocular lens power to produce refraction of approximately -8.00D. Typically patients elect for eventual bilateral surgery.

IOL Power Calculation in Complex Cases

Specific Methods to Use in Complex Cases

Third and fourth generation theoretical formulas, such as the Holladay II, SRK/T, and the Hoffer Q are generally preferred for complex cases. The regression formulas can induce undercorrection (e.g., SRK I or SRK II). In complex cases, multiple formulas should be evaluated and the surgeon should opt for a myopic result when in doubt.

Suggested Formulas Based Upon the Axial Length

As previously mentioned, if several formulas are available to the clinician, consider the following guidelines for formula selection based on axial length:
- Short eyes: AL <22.0 mm (8% of eyes): Holladay II, Hoffer Q, Haigis, and Hoffer-Collenbrander. These constitute 8-10% of cases.
- AL (axial length) between 22.00 and 24.0 mm (75% of eyes): The "average" formula, mean of the three formulas: Hoffer, Holladay and SKR/T, or the Holladay I.
- AL >24.0 mm (14% of eyes): the SRK/T or Holladay I formula.

High Hyperopia

Two main difficulties in measuring the axial length in axial hyperopia exist with the utilization of the correct ultrasound velocity (Hoffer has recommended using 1560 m/sec) and dealing with the errors induced by the ultrasound contact techniques in these short eyes.

Inadequate ultrasound velocity in short eyes is explained as follows: in general, biometers are calibrated for eyes with normal axial length and with a fixed proportion of solid and liquid media. These biometers use a mean ultrasound velocity of 1550-1555 m/sec, although the more recent biometric units utilize four marks and can measure each structure with its own velocity (anterior chamber 1532 m/

sec, lens 1641 m/sec, and vitreous 1432 m/sec), combining automatically these measurements and obtaining the axial length of the eye. In short eyes, the relation between the crystalline lens (solid media) is higher in relation to the liquid media (aqueous and vitreous) when compared to that of normal eyes and therefore the calculated axial length (AL) is shorter than the real AL as the global mean velocity is higher. Furthermore, contact biometry measurements may be inaccurate, due to the difficulty of the biometer finding the anterior capsular echo in shallow chambers. Finally, very short eyes are more prone to distortion created when gentle pressure is applied to the cornea.

In eyes with short axial lengths **(Figure 3A)**, the third generation formulas such as Holladay II and Hoffer-Q seem to provide the best results. While observing high refractive postoperative errors in extremely short eyes (<20.0 mm), Holladay discovered that the size of the anterior and posterior segments are not proportional and has suggested measurement of specific parameters that may lead to more accurate IOL power calculations. Assembling data from 35 international researchers, he concluded that about 20% of short eyes present a small anterior segment (nanophthalmic eyes); 80% present a normal anterior segment, however the posterior segment is typically abnormally short in both. This means that the formulas that predict a small anterior segment in short eyes will bring about an 80% error, leading to hyperopic errors of up to 5 diopters. The Holladay II formula utilizes the seven parameters previously described for IOL calculation: axial length, keratometry, ACD (anterior chamber depth), lens width, white-to-white corneal horizontal diameter, preoperative refraction, and age. This new formula has reduced 5 D errors to less than 1 D in the majority of eyes with high hyperopia.

The Use of Piggyback Lenses in High Hyperopia

Although the Holladay II and the Hoffer Q formulas offer significant advances in calculating IOL power in short eyes, implants higher than +40.0 diopters are not readily available, as they can induce significant spherical aberrations. In these patients requiring more than 40 diopters of IOL power, piggyback IOL implantation is indicated.

Gayton (1994) was the first to place two lenses in a single eye. He observed that placing multiple lenses in a single eye produces improved optical quality because there are less spherical aberration than with very high lens powers **(Figure 3B)**.

While measuring the position of piggyback lenses, Holladay observed that the anterior lens maintains its original position while the posterior lens moves backwards because of the distensible nature of the capsular bag. The total power of the piggyback IOL implantation is calculated more precisely with the Hoffer-Collenbrander (H-C), or with a modification of the Holladay II formula.

Gayton and Apple described the presence of interlenticular opacification (ILO) in endocapsular piggyback implantation. Histopathological examination revealed that the tissue consisted of retained/proliferative lens epithelial cells (bladder cells or pearls) mixed with lens cortical material which can be more aggressive when two acrylic optic IOLs are implanted into the capsular bag with a small capuslorhexis.

The following surgical maneuvers are recommended to prevent this complication: meticulous cortical cleanup, especially in the equatorial region; creation of a large continuous curvilinear capsulorhexis to minimize retention of equatorial lens epithelial cells; and insertion of the posterior IOL in the capsular bag with the anterior IOL in the ciliary sulcus. Finally, a combination of silicon and acrylic optic IOLs are recommended. To date, two cases of ILO have been described with piggyback IOL insertion outside the capsular bag in children (Villar-Kuri).

In conclusion, piggyback IOL implantation should be selected to patients needing more than +40.0 diopters of IOL power as calculated by the H-C or a modified Holladay II formula, and should be carefully implanted one in the capsular bag and one in the sulcus with different optic materials.

High Myopia

Results of cataract surgery in myopic and highly myopic eyes with implantation of low or negative power IOLs can be very successful. The use of the SRK/T formula showed good predictability in the calculation of the refractive target **(Figure 4)**. There are technical difficulties in performing the echobiometry of patients with high myopia, especially in presence of a posterior staphyloma. In these cases, irregular retinal echoes may not provide reliable measurements. Furthermore, a posterior staphyloma can be incoincidental with the macula, and the measurement obtained is not necessarily the correct axial length, as is the case with normal eyes.

In these patients it is most useful to perform a B ultrasound to identify the existence of a staphyloma and its relation with the macula. Equally important is to have an ultrasound probe with an incorporated fixation light. The patient is then asked to fixate at the light. In cases where fixation is difficult, it can be useful to ask the patient to fixate with the fellow eye another target.

In conclusion, it is suggested that in long and extremely long eyes, the IOL power calculation should be made after any previous corneal or vitreoretinal surgery has been ruled out, the patient has been out of contact lenses for a reasonable period of time (3 days for soft and 3 weeks for rigid gas permeable), reliable keratometric readings have been obtained, reliable and repeatable AL has been obtained with a B scan if a posterior staphyloma is present, and the SRK/T has been used as the preferred formula in these cases.

Determining IOL Power in Patients with Previous Refractive Surgery

IOL power calculation in patients who have had prior refractive surgery present a challenge as no universally accepted formula to calculate these patients' IOL power accurately exists. Furthermore, this population is psychologically resistant to wearing spectacles to correct residual ametropia and their expectations are unusually high. The primary challenge is that routine keratometry readings do not reflect the true central corneal curvature in these cases and may result in significant under or over correction. As a result, standard keratometric readings should not be used for IOL power calculations in these patients. Illustrations of B-scan ultrasonography in patients who have undergone excimer laser procedures, radial keratotomy, conductive keratoplasty, intra corneal segment rings, have had modifications to their corneal curvatures are depicted in (**Figures 6, 7, 8**).

One should make all efforts to obtain prior records and refractive information in order to utilize the refractive history method. This data is programmed into the selected formulas. The computer will then provide you with the power of the IOL to be utilized. IOL power calculation with multiple appropriate formulas is a suggested practice, including post refractive IOL calculators that are available on the internet *(www.iol.ascrs.org)*. Evaluating the mean of calculated IOL powers

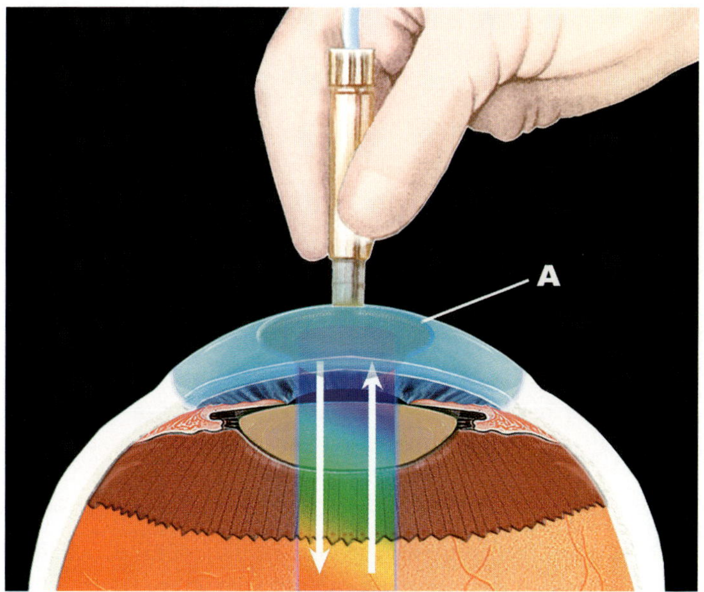

Figure 6: IOL power calculation after excimer laser procedure. In this group of patients there is a degree of variation in the results of the IOL power calculation. This is the result of the varying modification in the central curvature of the cornea after the central excimer laser ablation (A). (Art from Jaypee-Highlights Medical Publishers, Inc.)

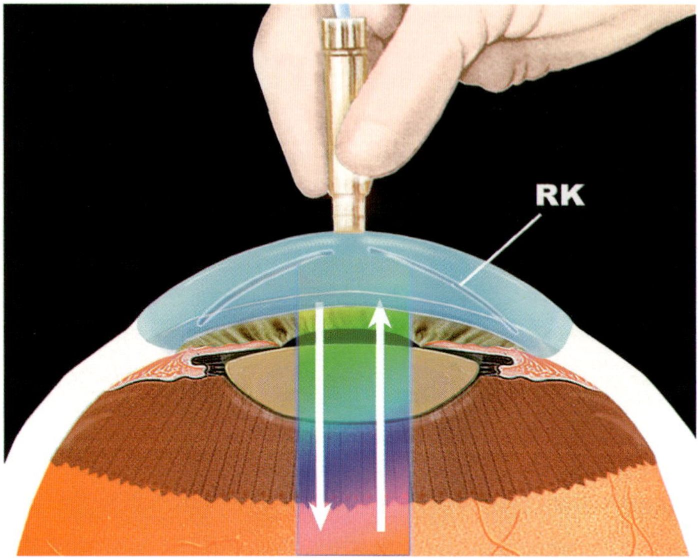

Figure 7: IOL power calculation in patients after radial keratotomy. Patients who have undergone previous radial keratotomy using an optical zone smaller than 4.0 mm, cannot have their central corneal curvature measured reliably with the standard keratometric methods. Axial length measurement may be done with the standard A scan ultrasonographic technique. (Art from Jaypee-Highlights Medical Publishers, Inc.)

can give the surgeon clues as to which IOL power to select. Of course, the final IOL power decision is a clinical one and the surgeon should use clues from the refractive outcome of the first eye if available. If there is no agreement and this is the first eye, consider leaning toward a higher IOL power.

Post Hyperopic LASIK

For previous hyperopic LASIK, the Haigis-L formula found in the IOL master and the ASCRS website, has proven to be very useful. One should take into account the induced negative spherical aberration induced by hyperopic LASIK, particularly in the event of large or consecutive treatments. I recommend using a neutral spherical aberration IOL in these cases, and avoiding aspheric IOLs. When calculating IOL power after multiple treatments, inputting the cumulative treatment typically works.

We also recommend the use of the central 3.0-mm corneal topography's flattest curve as an adjunctive keratometric method. Tomographic devices allow for measurement of the central corneal curvature, and new software can estimate the true net corneal power of a desired optical zone. Though Holladay suggests 4.5mm optical zone (OZ), other's have suggested use of 1.0 mm OZ in eyes with prior myopic refractive surgery (Intraocular lens power calculations after myopic

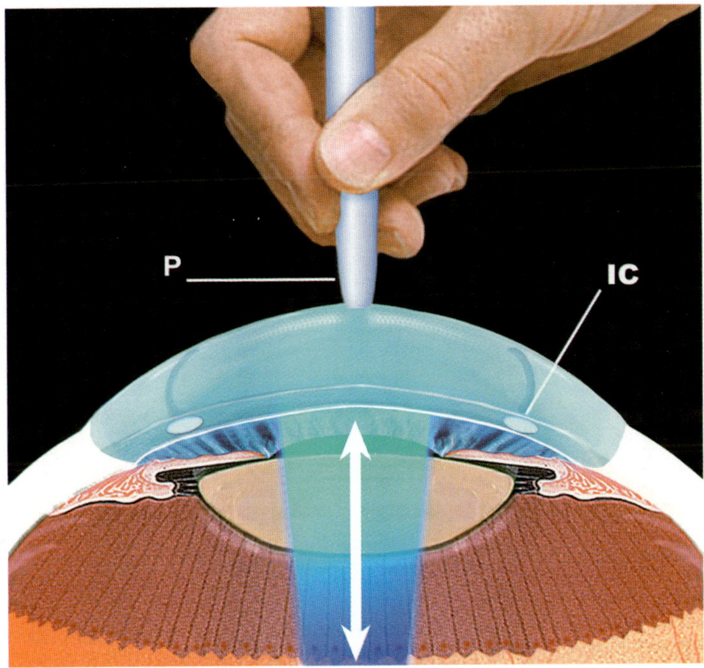

Figure 8: IOL power calculation after an intracorneal ring segment procedure. As with other refractive procedures on the cornea, this technique for correction of low myopia also modifies the corneal curvature. When the preoperative data is not available for the IOL power calculation by the history method, the central flattest K obtained by corneal topography is utilized for the IOL power calculation as the central corneal power. In this illustration we can see the ultrasound transducer (P) on the central cornea inside the area in which the Intracorneal Rings (IC) are placed. (Art from Jaypee-Highlights Medical Publishers, Inc.)

excimer laser refractive surgery: clinical outcomes and comparison of methods in 50 eyes Reeves et al., AAO 2007 poster). We recommend evaluation of multiple optical zones.

Intraoperative aberrometry is becoming more useful for post refractive IOL power calculation, though variation in outcomes still exists and this should be considered an adjunctive tool to the aforementioned described methodology. Interoperative aberrometry readings do add time to surgery, but this can be time well spent if the volume of post-refractive IOL eyes is appreciable, and may save time in the long run with chair time and enhancements.

Transient and diurnal fluctuations are common in eyes who have had previous radial keratotomy, particularly after IOL surgery due to stromal edema and relative effects of incision gape resulting in flattening of the cornea. The surgeons should counsel the patient to accept a transient fluctuation that can settle in 2-3 months. Enhancements should not be preformed during this period.

Methods Most Often Used

This section reviews the methods proposed to estimate the true power of the central cornea in eyes that have undergone corneal refractive surgery. The clinical history method and the contact lens method are well documented. As mentioned above, primary limitation includes determing the true optical central corneal power of the cornea using the present instrumentation available, as well as effective lens position. Keratometers and topographers measure the cornea too peripherally and miss the central, flat part of the cornea. The result is an overestimation of the corneal power that, when entered into the IOL power formula, produces an overly weak IOL power and thus a hyperopic refractive result. The advent of corneal tomographers that evaluate the central corneal curvature estimation as the posterior curvature, as well as advanced software allow surgeons to better estimate the true net central corneal power. The methods described herein are intended to better estimate the true power of the altered cornea.

Clinical History Method

Holladay proposed this method based on the idea that refractive surgery has changed the corneal power and that this refractive change must be substracted from the presurgical power of the cornea in order to estimate its present power. One needs to obtain:

- A preoperative average K reading (Kp).
- A preoperative spherical equivalent refractive error (Rp, before refractive corneal surgery).
- A postoperative spherical equivalent refractive error (Ro, after the eye has healed following refractive surgery and visual acuity has stabilized, prior to cataract formation).

To calculate the eye's estimated corneal power (K), use the Hoffer formula:

$$K = Kp + (Rp) - (Ro)$$

Remember to add algebraically and to change the sign when opening the second parenthesis. Vertex correcting refractions is no longer recommended.

Contact Lens Method

The contact lens method was first described by Ridley, later by Soper, and more recently published by Holladay. It was Hoffer who created a contact lens method formula. The method is based on the concept that, if a hard PMMA contact lens of known base curve (i.e. 36.00D) and known power (i.e., plano) is placed on the cornea and the refraction does not change, the effective power of the cornea must be 36.00 D. If the power is different from plano and/or the difference in refraction is not zero, the formula will calculate the power. This method is limited to those cataractous eyes with a minimum best corrected visual acuity of 20/80. The method will not work in eyes that are not able to be refracted.

You need to obtain:

- A hard PMMA (not RGP) contact lens with a base curve (B) close to the estimated K reading and with a known power (P, easier if plano).
- A bare manifest refraction without a contact lens (Rb).
- A manifest overrefraction with a contact lens (Rc).

To calculate the eye's estimated corneal power (K), use the formula:

$$K = B + P + Rc - Rb$$

Remember to add algebraically and vertex correction is no longer recommended.

Shammas' No History Method

In 2003, Shammas proposed a formula that only requires the postoperative average value obtained from a manual keratometer (Ko). To calculate the eye's estimated corneal power (K), use the formula: $K = 1.143 \times (Ko) - 6.8$.

Maloney Topography (Wang-Koch-Maloney) Method

Maloney originally described a formula later modified by Wang and Koch, now known as the modified Maloney method. Here, one needs to obtain only the postoperative simulated central K reading from the topographic unit (Kt) by placing the cursor on the center of the Axial Map of the Zeiss Humphrey Atlas topographer. This value is then converted back to the original anterior corneal power by multiplying the Axial Map central topographic corneal power by 376.0/337.5, which is the same as 1.114. An assumed posterior corneal power of 6.1 D is then subtracted from this product.

To calculate the eye's estimated corneal power (K), use the formula: $K = 376/ (337.5/Kt) - 5.5$, which is the same as, $(Kt \times 1.114) - 6.1$.

The Topography Method

When information is not available for the Clinical History Method, it has been recommended by Zacharias and Centurion, as well as by Torres and Suarez, that the keratometric reading be taken with the topography unit, using the flattest K found in the central 3mm of the corneal mapping.

Hoffer has suggested that after looking at the preceding methods, we should choose the lowest K reading from those you have calculated to use in the formula and then employ the Aramberri Double-K Method.

Double-K Method

A common source of postoperative error following refractive surgery is related to the ELP calculation. The ELP is the distance between the surfaces of the cornea (vertex) to the plane of the IOL. Third-generation formulas assume the K power and axial length to estimate the ELP. When using these formulas, very flat keratometric corneal power following refractive surgery will produce a false shallow postoperative ELP. As a result, the calculated IOL power will be underestimated, ensuing in a hyperopic error.

In 2003, Chamon described a double K method by using the preoperative and postoperative corneal power for IOL calculation after refractive surgery using the Holladay I formula. The preoperative K value was determined by topography, and the postoperative K value was determined by the clinical history method. A normal preoperative curvature (44.0D) is suggested for the preoperative value if not known, and the effective refractive power (EffRP) found in the EyeSys Corneal Analysis System is suggested for the postoperative value. As stated above, Aramberri went on to describe a double K method utilizing a modified SRK/T formula. Here, the preoperative K value was used to estimate the ELP and the post refractive K value, found by the clinical history method as described by Chamon, is used to calculate the IOL power with the vergence formula. The Holladay II formula also contains double K variables for post refractive surgical cases. If the preoperative K value is not known, Holladay recommends a K value of 43.86 D.

The Importance of Detecting Irregular Astigmatism

In addition to standard biomicroscopic and other testing, retinoscopy, corneal topography, tomography, whole eye wavefronts should be performed in all of complex cases. Many of these can aid in detection and assessment of irregular astigmatism. This is important because the irregular astigmatism may be contributing to the reduced vision, as well as the cataract. Irregular astigmatism may also be a limiting factor in the patient's visual potential.

The potential acuity meter (PAM), Super PinholeTM and hard contact lens trial are often helpful as secondary tests in determining the respective contribution to reduced vision by the cataract and the corneal irregular astigmatism **(Figure 9)**.

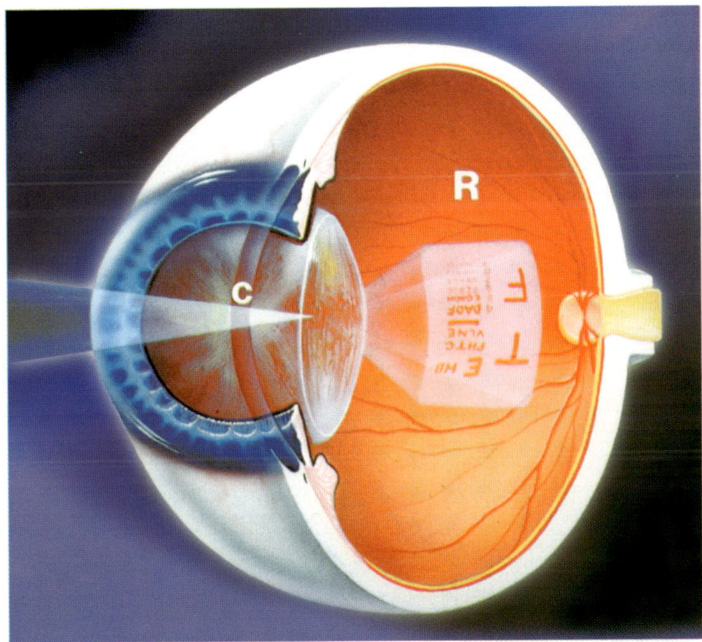

Figure 9: Concept of the Guyton-Minkowski potential acuity meter with cataractous lens (PAM). The beam of the projected Snellen chart is shown passing through a cataract (C) and forming the image of the chart on the retina (R). The beam of light can only strike the retina when it is able to pass through the opacities of the lens. With the chart successfully projected onto the retina, the patient can respond and we can determine the potential visual acuity as if the cataract was not there. Art from Jaypee-Highlights Medical Publishers, Inc.

The patient should also be informed that only symptoms related to the cataract will be eliminated. Any glare or night vision symptoms from other sources of aberration will essentially remain unchanged. In highly aberrated eyes, such as keratoconus where it is indicated to remove the cataract prior to corneal intervention, a reasonable approach is to assume a normal curvature (42.0-44.0D) for IOL calculations with the intention of preforming a staged procedure (lamellar or full thickness keratoplasty, intracorneal ring segments, corneal cross-linking). Ideally, the corneal procedure would be carried out first.

IOL Power Calculation in Pediatric Cataracts

Once a decision has been made to perform cataract surgery in a pediatric patient, the next consideration is the optical rehabilitation. For patients with monocular cataracts, aphakic spectacles are not practical. Before one year of age, use of contact lens rehabilitation is suggested in phakic eyes, after age 1 year, an IOL should be considered. In patients with bilateral cataracts, contact lens rehabilitation is recommended before 1 year of age. The unpredictable response and growth of an eye in a child less than one year of age may preclude selection of an IOL as a primary procedure in children.

The appropriate optical correction in patients with congenital cataracts has been a source of controversy for many years, due to axial growth with unstable and unpredictable outcomes **(Figure 10)**. It was considered impossible to predict such change and consequently, the accurate IOL power for every particular child. In addition, a pediatric lens capsule is prone to opacification of the posterior capsule in most cases, requiring a second operation when a posterior capsulotomy had to be performed in presence of an IOL.

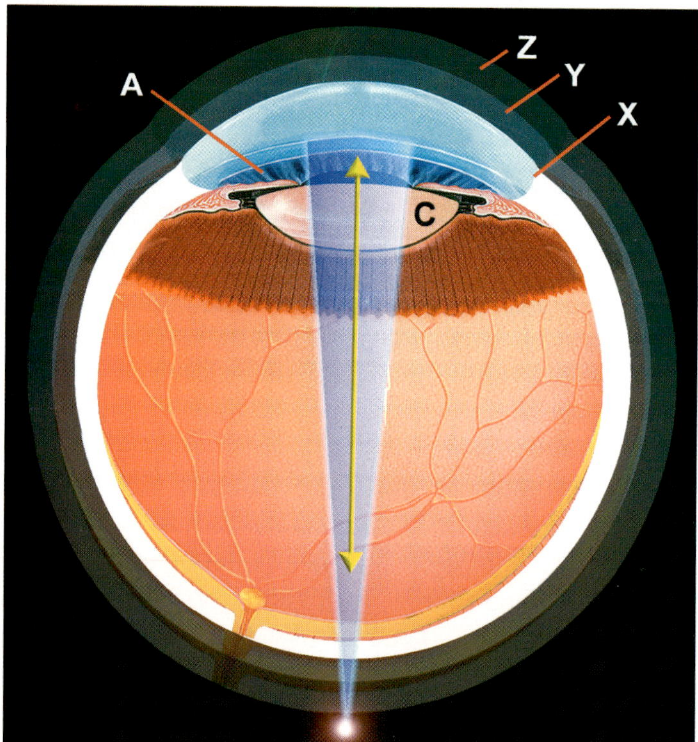

Figure 10: IOL power calculation in pediatric cataract. The growth of the globe is ecographically registered until young ages. However, the lens continues growing throughout the life of the individual. In normal circumstances, the anterior chamber (A) depth is reduced as the lens (C) increases in size. In this illustration we can see the changes in the size of the globe through the shaded images that outline the growth of the eye by stages. At birth, the eye measures approximately 17.5-mm; at three years of age it measures 21.8-mm (X), at ten years 22.5-mm identified in (Y), and in normal adulthood nearly 24-mm (Z). During IOL power selection, some surgeons do prefer to leave the child in a hyperopic stage (arrows) as emmetropia will be accomplished with the expected growth of the eye. Other surgeons prefer to aim for emmetropia for the prompt treatment of the associated amblyopia. (Art from Jaypee-Highlights Medical Publishers, Inc.)

The situation has now changed significantly. The previous failures with spectacles and contact lenses, the new developments in technology and surgical techniques, and the positive thinking of a new generation of surgeons has led us to implant posterior chamber IOLs in children. The development of improved medications to prevent and control inflammation, the introduction of posterior capsulorhexis, and better viscoelastics and IOLs, has allowed us to become more successful with IOL implantation in children.

Two primary methods of choosing an IOL power for pediatric patients are available: 1) to make the eye emmetropic at the time of surgery and thereby treat the amblyopia immediately after surgery by taking advantage of the improved potential visual acuity. This can be followed later by an IOL exchange or a secondary piggyback IOL implantation of a negative power IOL or any other means of treatment for the residual eventual myopia **(Figure 3-B)**. 2) Proceed with an incomplete (leaving the eyes hyperopic) correction of the eye at the time of surgery (the balance is treated with glasses or contact lenses), taking advantage of the trend toward emmetropization which will occur as the eye grows longer. As the eye grows in length with age (axial growth), the myopization that takes place in these postoperatively hyperopic eyes will trend toward emmetropia. This measure avoids myopic anisometropia which may lead to an undesirable surgical IOL exchange or other second surgical intervention. In the meantime, the temporary hyperopia is managed with standard spectacles or contact lenses. In IOL power calculation in children younger than 1 year, keratometry is difficult and fortunately less important because the values change very rapidly during the first six months of age. Thus, keratometry may be replaced by the mean adult average keratometry value of 42.50D (42.0-44.0D). Children with less than two years of age may be considered to be undercorrected by +3.00 D or to even +4.00 D; between three and four years of age to +3.00 D in those closer to three and +2.50 D in those closer to four. In ages six or seven, a targeted undercorrection of +1.00 D is recommended.

Additional considerations in selecting pediatric IOL powers include the age of the child, the refractive error of the fellow eye and the refractive error of the parents. Biglan calculates the lens power for the eye to achieve emmetropia using a SRK II formula. Aramberri recommends the use of the Third generation theoretical formulas. Biometric readings may be difficult to obtain in children. If the child has not had axial length determination or is uncooperative for preoperative studies, the axial length determination and keratometry are performed in the operating room after the child has been anesthetized. Lens power calculations are performed while the patient is being prepped and draped and the surgical microscope has been positioned. Finally, we recommended targeting 1.5 D or less of anisometropia.

IOL Power Calculation Following Vitrectomy

For the most part, IOL power calculation in eyes that develop a cataract following vitrectomy is straightforward. Intravitreal gas is reabsorbed and slowly replaced by aqueous humor. If silicone oil was used, once it is removed, aqueous fills the vitreous cavity. Since the refractive indices of aqueous and vitreous are identical (1.336), no corrections are needed in the IOL power calculation.

For patients who may undergo a silicone oil procedure at some point, it is wise to consider obtaining bilateral baseline axial length measurements by immersion A-scan biometry or by Optical Coherence Biometry -OCB (IOL Master). This category would include any patient with a prior retinal detachment, moderate to high axial myopia, proliferative vitreoretinopathy, proliferative diabetic retinopathy, acquired immune deficiency syndrome, giant retinal tear, or history of a perforating ocular injury **(Figure 11)**.

Eyes that have undergone complicated retinal detachment repair with silicone oil often require subsequent cataract surgery. Accurate A-scan biometry can be very difficult in these eyes because silicone oil has a slower sound velocity relative to vitreous and often produces strong sound attenuation. These factors may prevent the display of a high-quality retinal spike and can contribute to significant measurement errors. Therefore, it is best to use OCB to measure theses eyes whenever possible. Measurements can be made, without any special corrections, in phakic and aphakic eyes containing silicone oil. However, a large posterior subcapsular plaque or a dense nuclear cataract may make a reliable measurement impossible with this technique.

Two densities of silicone oil are presently in use, each of which has a slower sound velocity than vitreous (1532 m/sec). The 1000 centistokes (cSt) silicone oil has a sound velocity of 980 m/sec. The higher density 5000 cSt silicone oil produces a velocity of 1040m/sec. It is important to know which density of silicone oil is present in the vitreous cavity before A-scan biometry so that the correct velocity setting can be used.

For eyes containing silicone oil, A-scan axial length measurements are best carried out with the patient seated as upright as possible. This is especially important if the vitreous cavity is only partly filled with silicone oil. In the upright position, silicone oil is more likely to remain in contact with the retina during the examination. Because of its lighter density with the patient fully recumbent, the entire mass of silicone oil often shifts away from the retina, toward the anterior segment, leading to confusion as to the true position of the retinal spike.

If an incorrect sound velocity is used to measure the axial length of an eye containing silicone oil, the measurement displayed usually will be erroneously long. Measuring each component of the eye individually, using the correct corresponding sound velocity avoids errors and gives good approximation of the

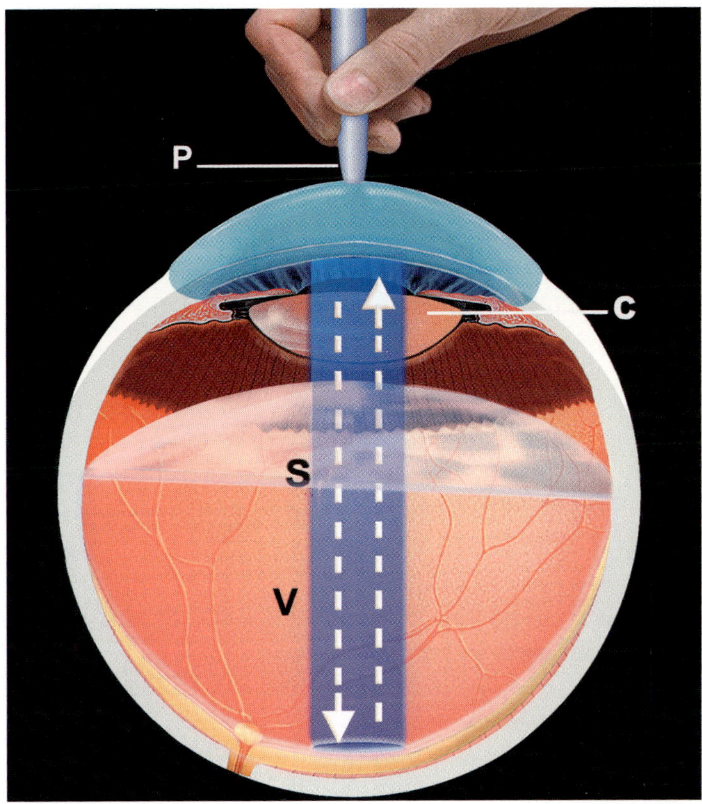

Figure 11: IOL power calculation in patients after vitrectomy procedure with silicone oil. Accurate A-scan biometry can be very difficult in eyes with silicone oil (S) in the vitreous cavity (V), since the oil has a slower sound velocity and often produces strong sound attenuation. These may prevent the display of a high-quality retinal spike and can contribute to significant measurement errors. Ultrasound probe (P). Crystalline lens (C). (Art from Jaypee-Highlights Medical Publishers, Inc.)

true axial length. Examples of sound velocities include anterior chamber depth at 1532 m/sec, crystalline lens thickness at 1641 m/sec, and vitreous cavity length at either 980 m/sec (for 1000 cSt silicone oil) or 1040 m/sec (for 5000 cSt silicone oil). Ideally, the biometer should have four electronic measuring gates and should allow the sound velocity to be modified when necessary. This allows for independent measurement of the individual components of the eye at the appropriate sound velocity. When the biometer provides only two gates and the sound velocities are not adjustable, a more complex approach is required.

If the silicone oil is to be removed at some point, standard IOL power calculations can be performed after the true axial length has been determined. However, if the silicone oil is to remain in the eye indefinitely, a power adjustment must be made to prevent significant postoperative hyperopia.

When silicone oil is placed in the vitreous cavity, a higher-power IOL is required to achieve the same refractive result. This is because the index of refraction for silicone is higher than that of normal vitreous. In addition, it is recommended that these patients receive a polymethylmethacrylate (PMMA) convex-plano lens; with the plano side oriented toward the vitreous cavity (and preferably over an intact posterior capsule). This approach prevents the silicone oil from altering the refractive power of the posterior surface of the IOL. The Holladay IOL Consultant software is very helpful for these cases as it has the ability to compensate for the different index of refraction of silicone oil compared to that of the vitreous.

The power that must be added to the original IOL calculation for a PMMA convex- plano IOL is determined by the following relationships:

$$\text{Power to be added} = \frac{Ns - Nv}{TALs - ACD} \times 1000$$

Ns is the refractive index of both 1000 cSt and 5000 cSt silicone oil (1.4034); Nv is refractive index of vitreous (1.336); TALs is the true axial length of an eye containing silicone oil in mm; and ACD is the measured anterior chamber depth in mm.

For an average-length eye in which the vitreous cavity is filled with silicone oil, the additional power needed for a convex-plano PMMA IOL is typically between + 3.0 D to + 3.5 D. For example, let's say the the true axial length (TALs) of an eye with 1000 cSt silicone oil filling the vitreous cavity is measured to be 25.17 mm. The anterior chamber depth is measured at 3.21 mm and the IOL power calculation calls for a plus 20.0 D convex-plano lens. In this circumstance, plus 3.07 D of additional IOL power must be added at the level of the capsular bag to compensate for the differing refractive index of silicone oil. This will result in the implantation of a plus 23.0 D lens.

If, however, removal of the silicone oil at a later date is anticipated, a possible alternative is to implant a plus 20.0 D convex-plano PMMA IOL in the capsular bag and a plus 3.0 D PMMA lens temporarily in the ciliary sulcus. The silicone oil and the ciliary sulcus lens could then be removed at the same time, thus avoiding a more complicated IOL exchange.

Meldrum, Aaberg, Patel, and Davis make the following recommendations:
- Measure the axial length using the velocity of sound in silicone oil.
- Calculate the IOL power to achieve emmetropia using the traditional formulas. To this IOL power, a correction factor must be added to obtain the IOL power to achieve emmetropia in silicone oil. The correction factors range from 2.79 D to 3.94 D, for axial lengths from 20 mm to 30 mm.

- Choose a convex-plano IOL if possible. If another type of lens is used, another or an additional correction factor must be added to obtain the total power of the IOL in the presence of silicone oil. For a convex-plano lens no additional correction factor is required with the aforementioned methodology.

For instance, let us suppose that a patient requires indefinite intraocular tamponade with silicone oil and develops a cataract. Using the traditional formulas, assuming that the IOL power is calculated to be 22.0D based on a measured axial length of 23 mm with the silicon oil settings. To this 22.0D we must add a correction factor of 3.64D (Meldrum et al) to correct for the axial length. Thus, for this patient a 25.5 D convex-plano lens should be implanted, with the plano side facing the vitreous cavity, to achieve emmetropia in the presence of silicone oil. No additional correction factor for the IOL design is necessary.

Conclusions

The aging population combined with trends toward lens refractive surgery is creating an increasing demand for lens surgery. Furthermore, the advent of premium technology, such as femto-phacosecond lasers for lens surgery, is creating a demand for premium outcomes. The methods described in this chapter will aid the surgeons with proper IOL calculations, the premise for excellent outcomes. Meticulous surgical technique and decision-making, combined with the proper IOL power selections will help surgeons achieve the desired result - happy patients.

Editorial Comment

Accurate biometric calculation is key for successful refractive solutions and in order to have our patients satisfied with the visual outcome of lens surgery. We have to know in advance our patient's everyday visual needs and surgical visual expectations. The surgeon must be acquainted with modern third and fourth generation formulas for calculating the power of the intraocular lens (IOL) and, if possible, use Partial Coherence Interferometry or Immersion Ultrasonography instead of Contact Biometry in order to determine the axial length with higher accuracy. Keratometry should be performed not only with manual and automated keratometers but also by corneal topography and tomography, which are especially useful in difficult cases such as irregular astigmatism and keratoconus.

In this chapter we describe in detail the factors that should be born in mind before calculating IOL power in complex cases or in those with previous refractive surgery.

Arnaldo Espaillat, MD

Recommended Readings

- Lu LW, Fine IH. Phacoemulsification in Difficult and Challenging Cases. New York: Thieme; 1999.
- Mendicute J, Aramberri J, Cadarso L, Ruiz M. Biometria, Formulas y Manejo de la sorpresa refractiva en la cirugia de catarata. Espana. Tecnimedia Editorial.2000.
- Shammas HJ. Intraocular Lens Power Calculations. Thorofare, NJ: Slack; 2004.

Recommended Internet Sites

- ASCRS post refractive IOL calculator (http://iol.ascrs.org/)
- Warren Hill IOL power calculations (http://doctor-hill.com/iol-main/iol_main.htm)
- iolocularmd.com

Bibliography

1. Aramberri J. Intraocular lens power calculation after corneal refractive surgery: Double K method. J Cataract Refract Surg 2003; 29: 2063-2068.
2. Boyd BF. Undergoing cataract surgery with a master surgeon: a personal experience. Highlights of Ophthalmol. Bi-monthly Journal, Volume 27, N° 1, 1999; 3.
3. Boyd, BF. The Art and Science of Cataract Surgery, 2001, 36-59
4. Brady KM., Atkinson CS., Kilty LA., Hiles DA: Cataract surgery and intraocular lens implantation in children. Am J Ophthalmol 1995; 120:1-9.
5. Buckley EG. Klombers LA., Seaber JH, et al: Management of the posterior capsule during intraocular lens implantation. Am J Ophthalmol 1993; 115:722-728.
6. Celikkol L, Pavlopoulos G, Weinstein B, et al. Calculation of intraocular lens power after radial keratotomy with computerized videokeratography. Am J Ophthalmol 1995; 120: 739-750.
7. Chen L, Mannis MJ, Salz JJ, et al. Analysis of intraocular lens power calculation in post-radial keratotomy eyes. J Cataract Refract Surg 2003; 29: 65-70.
8. Dahan E., Drusedan MUH.: Choice of lens and dioptric power in pediatric pseudophakia. J Cataract Refract Surg 1997; 23:618-23.
9. Gayton JL, Apple DJ, Peng Q, et al: Interlenticular opacification: Clinicopathological correlation of a complication of posterior chamber piggyback intraocular lenses. J Cataract Refract Surg 2000; 26:300-336.
10. Gimbel HV: Posterior continuous curvilinear capsulorhexis and optic capture of the intraocular lens to prevent secondary opacification in pediatric cataract surgery. J Cataract Refract Surg 1997; 23:652-656.
11. Gimbel HV., Basti S., Ferensowicz MA., DeBroff BM: Results of bilateral cataract extraction with posterior chamber intraocular lens implantation in children. Ophthalmology 1997; 104:1737-1743.
12. Grinbaum A, Treister G, Moisseiev J: Predicted and actual refraction after intraocular lens implantation in eyes with silicone oil. J Cataract Refract Surg 1996; 22:726-729.
13. Grusha YO, Masket S, Miller KM: Phacoemulsification and lens implantation after pars plana vitrectomy. Ophthalmology 1998; 105:287-294.
14. Hoffer KJ: Intraocular lens power calculation for eyes after refractive keratotomy. J Refract Surg 1995; 11:490-3.
15. Hoffer KJ: The Hoffer Q formula: A comparison of theoretic and regression formulas. J Cataract Surg 1993; 19:700-711.
16. Hoffer KJ: Ultrasound velocities for axial length measurement. J Cat Refract Surg 1994; 20:554-562.
17. Holladay JT: Intraocular lens power in difficult cases. In: Atlas of Cataract Surgery. Masket S, Crandall A. (ed) Martin Dunitz, 1999, 19:147-158.

18. Holladay JT., Gills JP, Leidlein J, Cherchio M: Achieving emmetropia in extremely short eyes with two pig-gyback posterior chamber intraocular lenses. Ophthalmology 1996; 103:1118-1123.
19. Holladay JT. Consultations in refractive surgery. Refract Corneal Surg 1989; 5: 203.
20. Holladay JT. Standardizing constants for ultrasonic biometry, keratometry and intraocular lens power calcu-lations. J Cataract Refract Surg 1997; 23: 1356-1370.
21. Koch D, Wang I. Calculating IOL power in eyes that have had refractive surgery. J Cataract Refract Surg 2003; 29: 2039-2042.
22. Kora Y., Shimizu K, Inatomi M, et al: Eye growth after cataract extraction and intraocular lens implantation in children. Ophthalmic Surg 1993; 24:467-475.
23. Lyle WA, Jin GJC: Intraocular lens power prediction in patients who undergo cataract surgery following previous radial keratotomy. Arch Ophthalmol 1997; 115:457-461.
24. McCartney DL, Miller KM., Stark WJ, et al: Intraocular lens style and refraction in eyes treated with silicone oil. Arch Ophthalmol 1987; 105:1385-1387.
25. Maeda N, Klyce SD, Smolek MK, McDonald MB.Disparity between keratometry-style reading and corneal power within the pupil after refractive surgery for myopia. Cornea 1997; 16: 517-524.
26. Meldrum LM., Aaberg TM, Patel A, et al: Cataract extraction after silicone oil repair of retinal detachments due to necrotizing retinitis. Arch Ophthalmol 1996; 114:885-892.
27. Milaukas AT, Marney S. Pseudo axial length increase after silicone lens implantation as determined by ultrasonic scans. J Cataract Refract Surg 1988; 14: 400-402.
28. Olsen T, Nielsen PJ. Immersion vs contact in the measurement of axial length by ultrasound. Acta Ophthal-mol 1989; 67: 101-102.
29. Olsen T, Thim K, Corydon L,: Theoretical versus SRK I and SRK II calculation of intraocular lens power. J. Cataract Refract Surg 1990; 16:217-225.
30. Rajan MS, Keilhorn I, Bell JA. Partial coherence laser Interferometry vs conventional ultrasound biometry; outcomes analysis. Eye 2002; 16: 552-556.
31. Sanders DR, Retzlaff J, Kraff MC, et al: Comparison of the SRK/T formula and other theoretical and regres-sion formulas. J Cataract Refract Surg 1990; 16(3):341-346.
32. Shammas HJ. A comparison of immersion and contact techniques for axial length measurements. J Am Intraocul Implant Soc 1984; 10: 444-447.
33. Yang S, Lang A, Makker H, et al. Effect of silicone sound speed and IOL thickness in pseudophakic axial length corrections. J Cataract Refract Surg 1995; 21: 442-446.
34. Zacharias W., Centurion, V: Biometry and the IOL calculation for the cataract surgeon: Its importance. Faco Total 2000; 66-88.
35. Zaldivar R, Schultz MC, Davidorf JM, et al. Intraocular lens power calculations in patients with extreme myopia. J Cataract Refract Surg. 2000; 26: 668-674.

4 | Dynamics of Nucleus Emulsification

AK Grover, MD
Shaloo Bageja, MS

The aim of phacoemulsification is to emulsify the central core of the lens or the nucleus using minimum possible phaco energy and surgical maneuvers producing the least possible trauma to the intraocular structures viz the cornea, the iris and the posterior capsule.

To accomplish a successful procedure the surgeon should be well versed with anatomy of the nucleus, instruments and the dynamics of the emulsification process in order to perform the surgery safely and quickly.

APPLIED ANATOMY

The lens is divided into four parts from the surgeon's point of view - central core, epinucleus, cortex and capsule **(Figure 1)**.

As age advances the peripheral cortical fibers are pushed centrally and with decrease in water content, the density of the central nucleus increases. As nucleus progresses from softness to hardness there is color change from transparent to white or greenish yellow, yellow, amber brown and then black. Epinucleus also undergoes sclerosis. With increase in density of the nucleus, the densest part is placed posteriorly and it is important to have 90% depth of the trench in the nucleus before cracking is attempted as the fibers are leathery and difficult to separate.

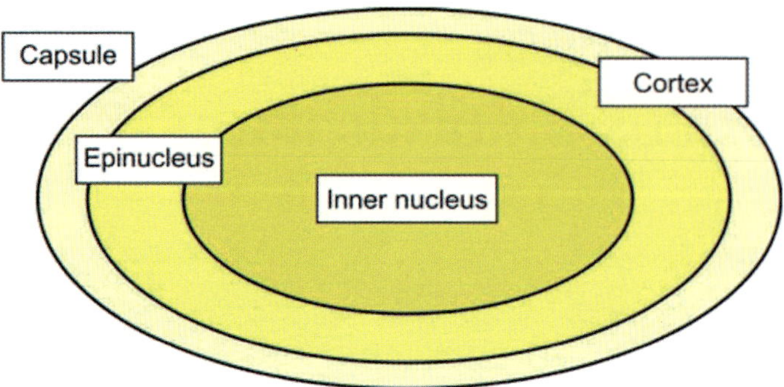

Figure 1: Surgical anatomy of the crystalline lens.

INSTRUMENTS

1. Phaco tip
2. Chopper

Phaco Tips

Various types of tips are available like the standard, microflow, Kelman and the Kelman flare tip. Angulation of the tip may be 15°, 30°, 45° and 0°. The 0 and 15° tips have greater occlusion capacity, the 45° one has greater cutting capacity while the 30° tip is a compromise of the two features.

The *standard tip* is the most commonly used tip. It has a 0.9 mm inner and 1.1 mm outer diameter. The microflow tip has an internal diameter ranging from 0.45 to 0.6 mm. It is usually recommended for soft to moderate hard cataracts as the smaller surface area of the tip does not provide a high holding power. It is not recommended for the hard cataracts.

Kelman tip with downward angulation is ideal for hard cataracts but there may be chances of a posterior capsule rupture in the hands of the beginners. They should change to a regular tip after the trenching. *Kelman flared tip* has a wider distal area, transmits more power and is used for harder cataracts.

Choppers/Sinskey Hook

The Sinskey hook or chopper is a valuable second instrument for phacoemulsification. It consists of a handle, horizontal and a vertical part. They can be blunt or sharp tipped choppers or an elongated sinskey. It is used for stabilizing the globe, rotation of the nucleus, splitting and chopping of the nucleus and also aids in feeding the nuclear fragments into the tips.

NUCLEUS EMULSIFICATION

Techniques

The nucleus emulsification can be performed adopting various techniques:
A. Divide and conquer
B. Stop and chop
C. Flip and chip
D. Direct chop or
E. Akahoshi Prechop

However, all these techniques, involve some basic phacodynamics which is dealt with here.

Basic Dynamics of Nucleus Phacoemulsification

The emulsification of nucleus requires ultrasonic power which is produced by the piezoelectric crystal in the hand piece. It is created by the interaction of the frequency and stroke length. Frequency is defined as the speed of the tip. It vibrates at a specific frequency when it is excited by an electrical field. The electrical energy creates an ultrasonic vibration of frequency varying from 28,000 to 60,000 Hz which is transmitted to the tip as longitudinal vibration. The mechanical energy generated contributes to emulsification of the nucleus. Phaco power implies the extent of excursion of the phaco tip. Most machines operate in 2-4 crystals. Longer excursions means greater impact on the nucleus and greater energy generation. All machines provide 0-100% power and the required power is chosen from the panel.

Power Modulations in Phacoemulsification

The phaco surgeons should be aware of all the power modulations, utilizing these as one is able to emulsify hard cataract using low energy without causing any damage to endothelial cells and iris.

Phaco machine has been provided with two different modes i.e *surgeon mode* and *panel mode*. In surgeon mode, the delivery of power is varied from zero to maximum set power depending on the position of the foot pedal. While in panel mode, the maximum power is delivered as soon as the surgeon presses the foot pedal. The surgeon mode is usually preferred by the phaco surgeons as power can be varied according to the density of the nucleus in the part being emulsified, as we are aware the nucleus is not homogenous in density.

Pulse Phaco

In pulse mode, the pulse of fixed energy is followed by a gap of off time of equal duration **(Figure 2)**. The frequency of pulse is fixed but the power can be varied depending upon the position of the foot pedal. As soon as the surgeon switches to extreme position of foot pedal, the pulse mode is transformed to linear mode. The interval between the pulses allows the vacuum to build up and a good hold is achieved. Different machines have different set of pulses. As low as 2-6 pulses are adequate for nucleus emulsification.

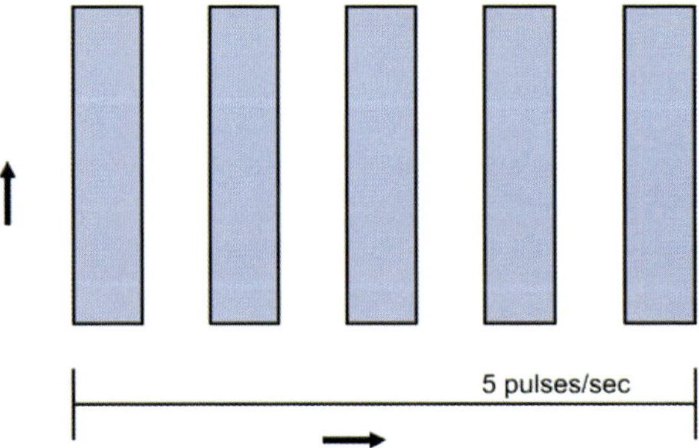

Figure 2: Pulse mode, showing 5 pulses/sec, each pulse being 100 msec in duration.

Duty Cycle

It is the percentage of time phaco is on to total phaco time. In standard pulse mode, there is duty cycle of 50% i.e 5 pulses/ second meant that each pulse interval is 200 msec, of which 100 msec is phaco on time while 100 msec is phaco offtime. With availability of newer software, the duty can be further reduced to 33% or 25%. Once chosen pulses/sec and duty cycle remain constant as set on the panel regardless of the foot pedal position.

Burst Mode

In the burst mode maximum preset power is delivered at intervals, varied according to the foot pedal position. The frequency of phaco bursts increases with depression of footpedal and delivers continuous energy at full excursion of the foot pedal **(Figure 3)**.

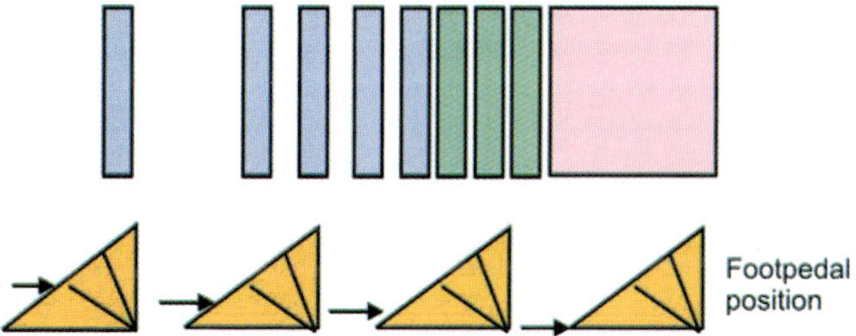

Figure 3: Burst mode. Maximum preset power is delivered each time. Frequency of the burst varies depending upon the position of the foot pedal. On full pedal depression, the power delivery becomes continuous.

Variations of Burst Duration

Use shorter duration of 25 msec for softer cataracts and larger duration of 50 msec or even more for harder cataracts.

Hyperpulse Mode

This power modulation allows the surgeon to vary the duty cycles depending upon the density of the cataract. In soft cataract, one can have low duty cycle of 15-20% and low phaco energy such as 30%. While in harder cataracts, phaco-energy is increased to 50% with duty cycle of 25-33%. This allows a large cooling time after each pulse of power, making it a cold phaco **(Figure 4)**.

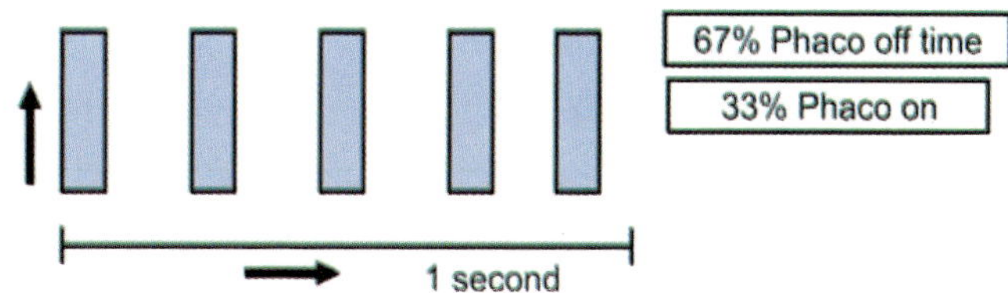

Figure 4: Hyperpulse mode with a duty cycle of 33% phaco on time.

Whitestar

The whitestar technology has 10 preset programs regarding hyperpulse/duty cycle settings. These settings are defined by the fixed period of phaco on and phaco off intervals, which a surgeon can choose. The lowest duty cycle available is 4 milliseconds of phaco-on followed by 24 milliseconds of phaco off time.

Variable Whitestar

In this mode, surgeon can adjust four different whitestar settings through the depression of the foot pedal in position 3. At the beginning of footposition 3, one can get lower duty cycle settings but as the foot pedal is depressed, one can shift to higher duty cycles mode. This allows the surgeon a bimodal linear increase in phaco power and duty cycle and thus enhancing the phaco power and cutting when needed.

Occlusion Mode

This mode allows the application of different phaco settings before and after tip occlusion. On occlusion, one should have a higher duty cycle, higher power and lower aspiration flow rate. When the probe is occluded by the nuclear fragment, vacuum rises beyond the prefixed settings, the phaco power automatically rises for greater cutting efficiency and the flow rate decreases. This avoids the postocclusion surge. Once the occlusion is cleared, the settings return to their original levels.

The surgeon can utilize the various power modulations at different steps of surgery in achieving successful surgery. Continuous mode with phaco energy of 50-60% with low vacuum settings is used for sculpting. Microbursts with high vacuum provides strong occlusion which can also be used for direct chopping. Hyper pulse mode is used for quadrant removal with a settings of 30-50 pulses/sec with a 33% duty cycle. This increases the followability, due to rapid cycling between phaco on and phaco off time. Repulsive forces are reduced and chattering of pieces in the anterior chamber is avoided.

Infiniti

In this mode the number of maximum pulses has increased to 100 pulses/sec from maximum of 15 pulses/sec in legacy. The surgeon can also preset dutycycle from 5% to 95%, earlier being fixed at 50%. This change gives the surgeon complete control over the phaco-on and phaco-off time.

Neosonix

Neosonix with Advantec (Legacy, Alcon surgical) provides the additional low frequency oscillatory energy to the ultrasound. The oscillations can be varied upto 2 degrees at 120 HZ. The low frequency oscillations can be used alone at low frequency to burrow into the nuclear fragment or in combination with phaco power.

Sonic Mode

Sonic (Staar wave, Staar surgical) uses sonic rather than ultrasonic energy. It fragments the nucleus without generating heat. Its frequency varies from 40 to 400 Hz in sonic range. The sonic phaco probe and tip can be utilized for sonic and ultrasonic mode. The surgeon can alternate between the two modes or can use them simultaneously.

OZil Torsional Mode

OZil IP Torsional ultrasound, which is unique to the INFINITI Vision System (Alcon Laboratories, Inc.), has been proven to remove all grades of cataract more effectively than traditional phacoemulsification with longitudinal ultrasound. OZil Torsional ultrasound moves the phaco tip in a shearing motion for nuclear disassembly, in contrast to the forward-and-backward jackhammer action of the phaco tip in traditional longitudinal phacoemulsification. The shearing motion is more effective at emulsifying nuclear material because each stroke of the phaco tip consumes material. In longitudinal ultrasound, only the forward motion of the phaco tip fragments the nucleus. In fact, the backward movement of the phaco needle is considerably at some point disadvantageous, because it tends to release the needle's hold on the fragment. Because OZil Torsional ultrasound is twice as efficient as longitudinal ultrasound, it requires less total energy to fully emulsify a nucleus.

Stellaris System

The Stellaris technology (Bausch & Lomb), was engineered to advance longitudinal phaco by increasing its stroke by 25% to improve mechanical cutting and utilizing low frequency (28.5 kHz) to optimize cavitational energy.

The ultrasonic power works as the interaction of four distinct components: mechanical impact of the tip, cavitation, formation of a fluid wave and an acoustical wave. The Stellaris was designed also for techniques including bimanual and 1.8-mm microcoaxial phaco.

TRENCHING

Emulsification is performed by the phaco tip which operates like a jack hammer, the to and fro movement of the tip and by the cavitation phenomenon. It is important to introduce the phaco probe at an angle to sculpt the surface of the nucleus. If it is placed parallel to the surface it would vibrate to and fro without sculpting.

The trenching is started from the center of the nucleus and movement is made towards the capsulorhexis margin. The forward movement consisting of shaving action, should be kept short of the capsulorhexis margin, thus avoiding injury to iris **(Figures 5 and 6)**. The tip should not be buried more than half the width of the tip to avoid occlusion of the tip. The phaco power is adjusted to achieve a smooth sculpting without pushing the nucleus and avoiding generation of excessive intraocular energy. The power should not be too less as it may push the nucleus and exert stress on the zonules.

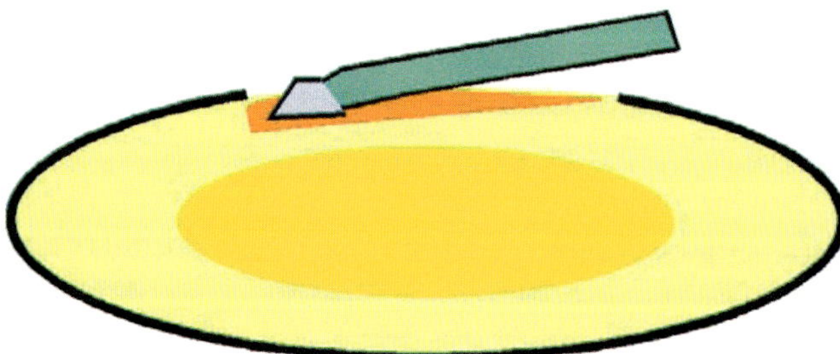

Figure 5: Shaving action of the probe, the trench is kept short of the capsulorhexis margin.

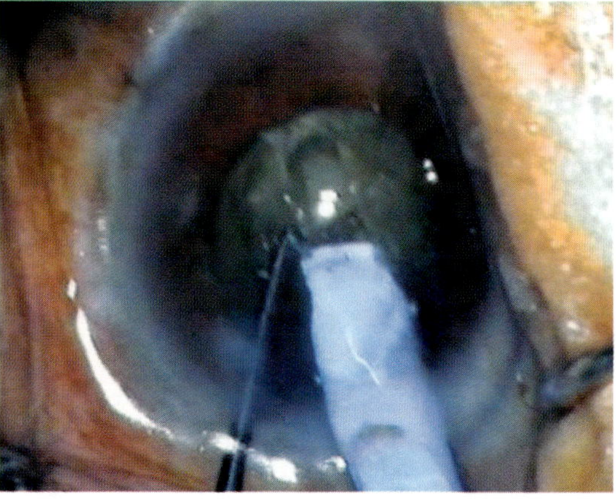

Figure 6: A photograph of the trench created in the nucleus. The trench is short of the capsulorhexis margin.

The power is determined by:
1. The density of the nucleus
2. Amount of tip engaged
3. Linear velocity of the tip

The phaco is kept in a linear mode during trenching for better control as the nucleus is not homogenous and has a variable density. The nucleus is less dense in the periphery and therefore the power requirement is low initially. It is increased in the central part of nucleus depressing the foot pedal and as the center of the nucleus is passed the foot pedal is raised to decrease the delivery of power. On the return, there should be no power or aspiration. The phaco surgeons should use low magnification as it provides wider field of view and allows him to assess the nuclear movements while sculpting and them to assess the depth and width of the trench. As he goes deeper, the surgeon can go beyond the capsulorhexis margin due to the available protective layer of epinucleus.

Width of the Groove

The width of the trench should be approximately two tip diameter. The width can vary according to the density of the nucleus. A wide groove in soft cataract is not required as the second instrument will not have much support to facilitate nucleus rotation. On the other hand, a hard cataract will require a wider trench. Initially a central groove is made and the trench is then widened by tilting the tip with bevel facing towards the center **(Figure 7)**.

One should be cautious to maintain an adequate width of the groove posteriorly even if it is adequate anteriorly. Sometimes even though the sleeve may fit into the trench, it may be pushing the nucleus, applying stress on the zonules.

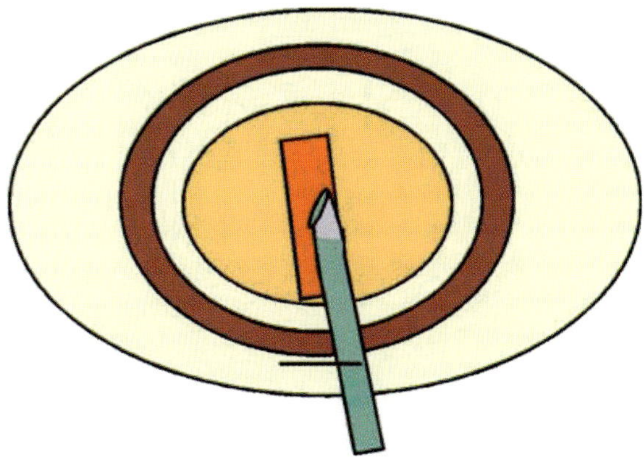

Figure 7: Trench is behind widened by tilting the tip of the probe with bevel facing towards the center.

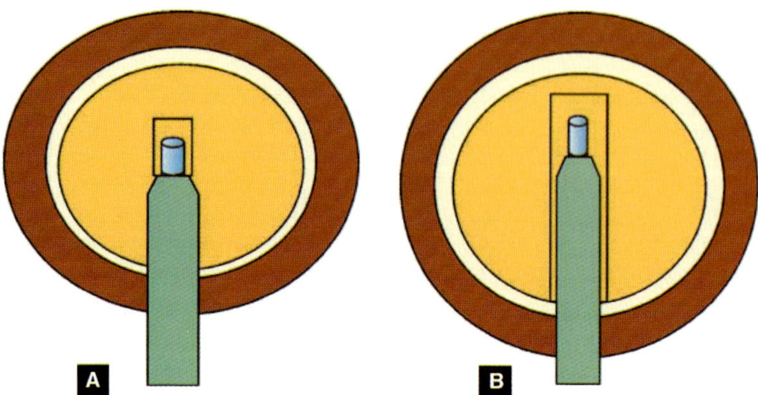

Figures 8A and B: (A) Inadequate width of the trench as sleeve just fits into trench,
(B)   Showing an adequate width of the trench.

It may in such a situation, be necessary to widen the groove posteriorly to avoid stress on the zonules **(Figures 8A and 8B)**. If the trench is not widened and the surgeon tries to push the tip by increasing the ultrasound power there may be unfavorable outcomes including zonular tears and posterior capsule rupture.

Peripheral Groove

The golden ring of hydrodelineation is an important landmark for the peripheral limit. The trench should be deeper centrally than peripherally.

Depth

The required depth of the trench will vary depending upon the density of the nucleus. Harder cataracts have a large nucleus and will require a deep trench which should follow the posterior convexity of the nucleus.

The required depth of trench can be assessed according to the following factors:

1. *Preoperative assessment:* Depending on the density of the nucleus.
2. *Intraoperative:*
    a.   Thin epinucleus suggests large nucleus.
    b.   *Size of the delineation ring:* Large ring indicates large nucleus.
    c.   Golden ring formation indicates a softer nucleus with small central core.

It is important for a surgeon to assess the depth of trench which can be done by:

Red reflex: The red reflex is visible peripherally in the moderate density nucleus but the reflex gets brighter as the thickness of the nucleus is reduced by sculpting.

Parallax technique: It is especially used for posterior cortical or subcapsular cataract. On moving the nucleus from side to side the movements of the posterior opacities relative to the base of the groove is assessed. The opacities will move less as trench is deepened.

NUCLEUS ROTATION

The trench is widened and deepened with multiple strokes. The nucleus can be rotated single handedly or bimanually to make the sub incisional nucleus accessible for further trenching.

The rotation of the nucleus is based on the principles of torque. The rotation is achieved if the lever arm is long and force applied is minimum.

$$Torque = Force \times Lever\ arm$$

As we know the initial groove is longer at 6 o'clock postion than at 12 o'clock position.

Figure 9 shows the nucleus rotation with a spatula through the side port. At point X, if the nucleus is rotated clockwise the force required is less as the lever arm is long but if one rotates anticlockwise at point Y, the required force will be double. The spatula should be placed against the hardest part of the nucleus, otherwise the instrument may penetrate into the nucleus rather than rotating it.

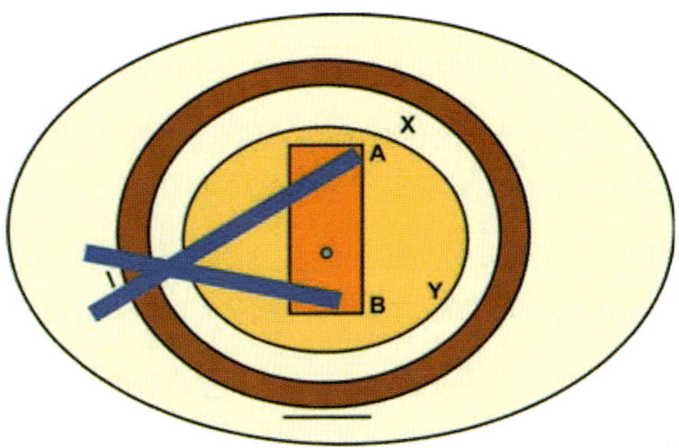

Figure 9: At position X, the force required for dialing is less as the distance from the axis of rotation is more as compared to the position Y.

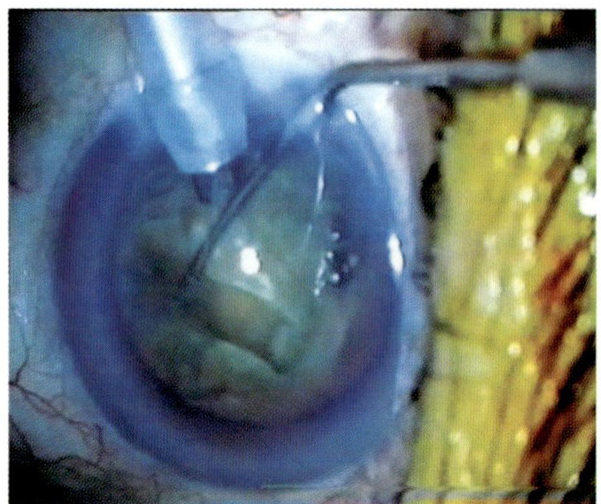

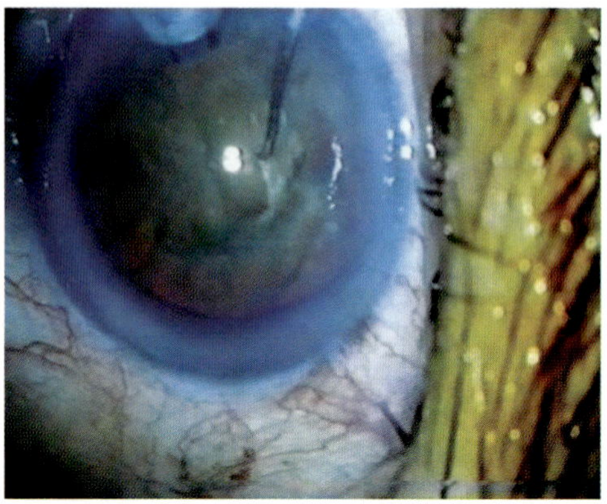

Figure 10A: Rotating the nucleus by placing the dialer in the trench.

Figure 10B: Sculpting is continued after rotation to complete the trench.

After 180° rotation, trench is enlarged at 6 o'clock position. The sculpting is started superficially and continuing the shaving action, a trench of uniform depth is achieved (**Figures 10A and B**).

NUCLEUS ROTATION WITH PHACO TIP

The phaco tip is embedded into the nucleus with a short burst of phaco and once the vacuum seal is obtained, phaco tip is used to manipulate the nucleus. It is important to ensure that the bevel of the tip is completely embedded into the nucleus to achieve a vacuum seal.

NUCLEUS CRACKING

After achieving an adequate depth trench, the nucleus needs to be split into two halves. One should apply forces in an appropriate direction to avoid stress on the zonules. The splitting of the nucleus will depend upon its density, the distance between the points where forces are to be applied and the depth of the groove.

The application of the forces should be near to each other, in order to prevent unnecessary stress on the nucleus (**Figures 11A andB**). The two instruments either chopper or Sinskey hook and phaco probe should be kept near the bottom of the trench and should be close. The force applied is in the opposite directions so that center of the nucleus depresses backward and the peripheral part lifts upward. If the movement of the nucleus is not such it indicates that either the trench is superficial or the placement of the nucleus is not proper.

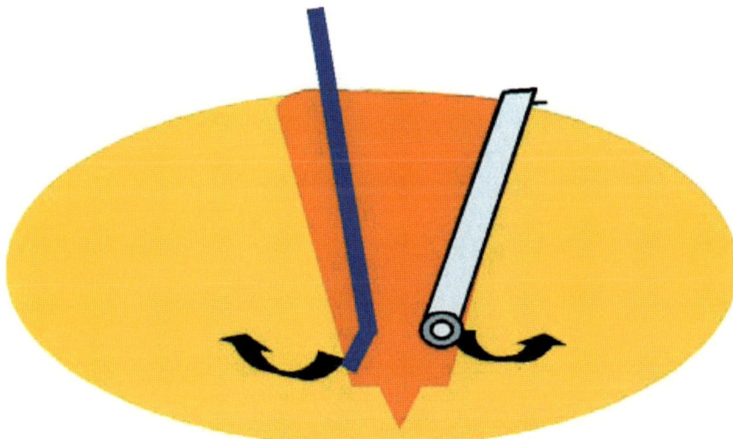

Figure 11A: Correct placement of two instruments at the bottom of the trench and forces are applied in opposite direction.

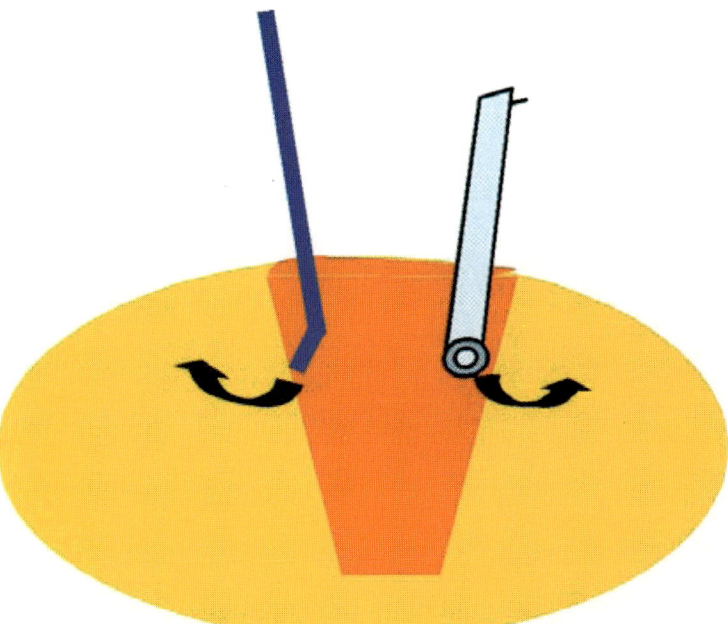

Figure 11B: Incorrect superficial placement of instruments.

If splitting is incomplete, it is necessary to split in the periphery or complete it after rotating the nucleus **(Figures 12A and B).** In harder leathery nucleus of brown and black cataracts it is necessary to split at multiple points in order to get a complete separation.

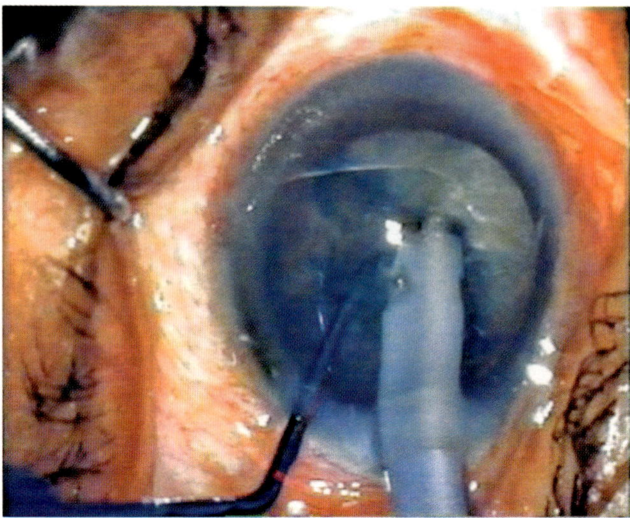

Figure 12A: Splitting of the nucleus into two halves using the phaco probe and the dialer.

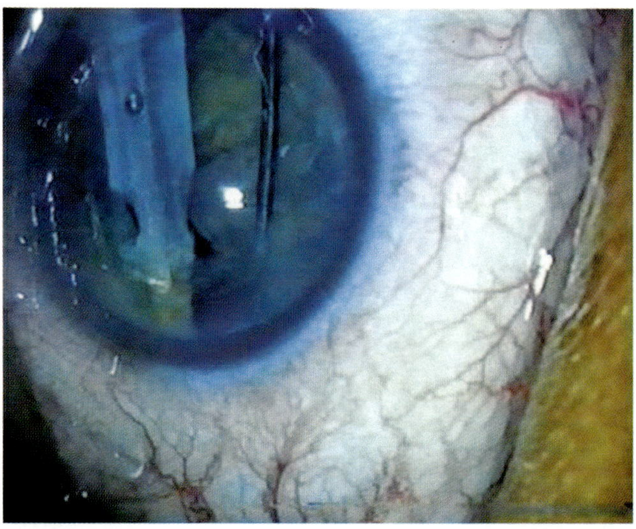

Figure 12B: If splitting is incomplete, it is necessary to continue splitting in the peripheral part of the trench.

CHOPPING

It is a technique where the nucleus is divided into smaller pieces with a chopper or sinskey hook. Chopping may be used for direct chopping of the entire nucleus or it may be used for chopping of the halves or quadrants or smaller pieces of the nucleus. Chopping can be done using a central, peripheral or a modified peripheral approach.

DIRECT CHOP OF NUCLEUS

The principle for application of forces are same. The phaco tip is embedded in the densest part of the nucleus, creating a vacuum seal by high vacuum and higher power settings, thus stabilizing the nucleus. The burst/ panel mode is preferred. It is then lifted, the chopper is introduced peripheral to the phaco probe in line with it **(Figure 13A)**. The chopper must be directed posteriorly at a sufficient depth, towards the center of the globe. It is then moved towards the phaco probe. The phaco probe and the chopper are then moved in the opposite directions, splitting the nucleus into two halves **(Figure 13B)**. This technique is not preferred in the softer cataracts as the probe can go through and through. This technique uses less phaco energy and is faster.

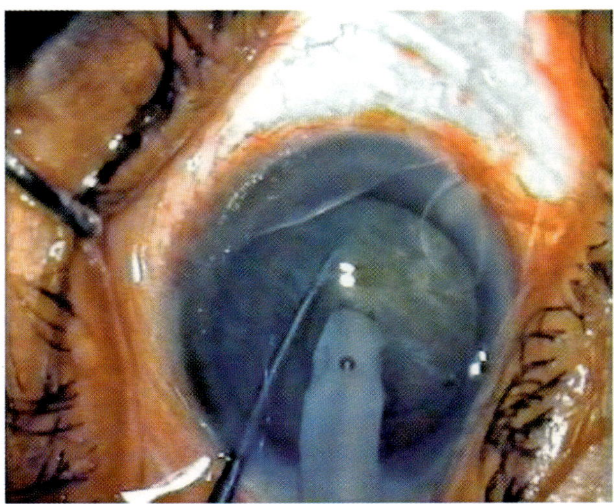

Figure 13A: Direct chopping of the nucleus. The phaco probe is embedded in the nucleus using a burst of energy and a high vacuum.

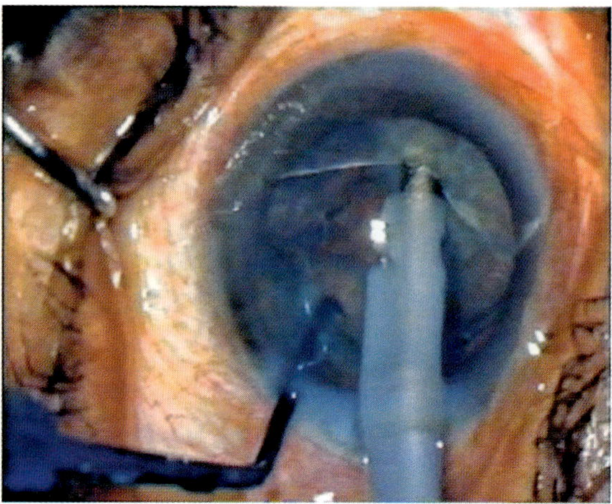

Figure 13B: Chopping being performed, with a sideward movement splitting the nucleus into two halves.

Peripheral Chop

The chopper is introduced horizontally under the capsulorhexis margin upto the periphery of the nucleus, avoiding injury to rhexis margin **(Figure 14A)**. The nucleus half is positioned horizontally and is engaged by the phaco probe giving a burst of energy in the center of the piece **(Figure 14B)**. Once the vacuum is built up, the nucleus is drawn centrally. The chopper is rotated vertically, engages the nucleus in the periphery in the line of the phaco probe and is pulled towards the phaco probe. When it reaches near the tip it is moved sideways, splitting the nucleus from the periphery to its center.

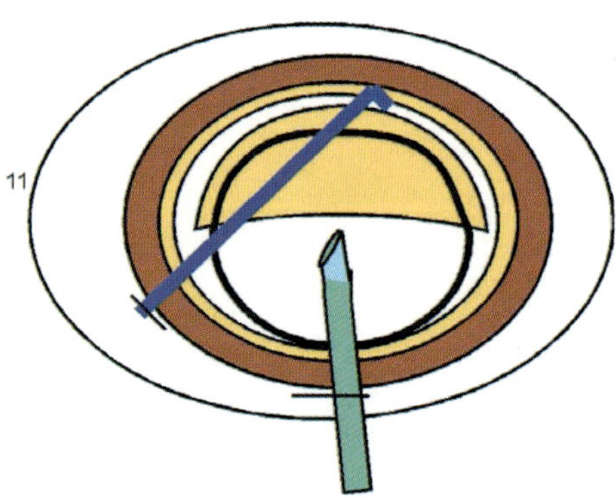

Figure 14A: Peripheral chopping. Placement of chopper underneath the capsulorhexis margin outer to the periphery of the nucleus.

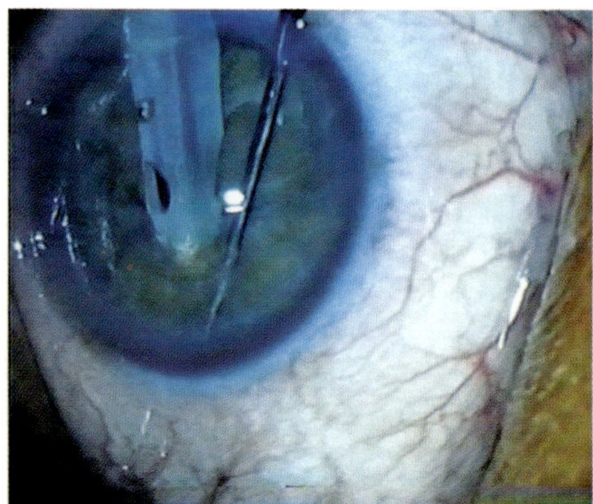

Figure 14B: Peripheral chopping of the nuclear half.

Central Chop

The central chop involves splitting of the fibers rather than cutting. It can be performed either by a Sinskey hook or a sharp chopper. The probe is embedded in the nucleus, vacuum hold is created and the chopper is placed just peripheral to the phaco probe and to the left to it **(Figure 15A)**. The chopping is performed by a posterior pressure with the chopper, at the same time pulling the chopper sideways or by pulling them both in the opposite directions **(Figures 15B and C)**.

If the chopper is not placed properly, there will be a rotation of the nucleus.

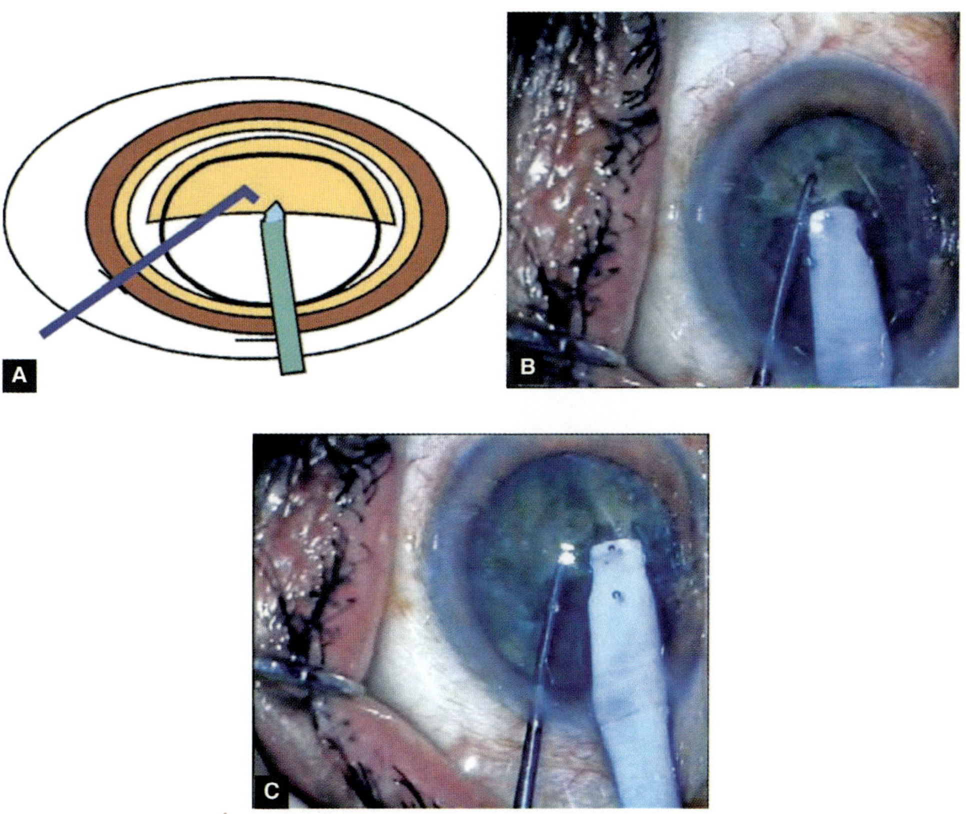

Figure 15A to C: (A) Placement of chopper in the center of the nuclear fragment to the left of the phaco probe which engages the nuclear fragment, (B) The position of the chopper after the nucleus is engaged. A backward pressure is applied by the chopper, (C) The two instruments move sideways to split the nucleus half.

Modified Peripheral Chop

This approach utilizes the advantages of both the central and peripheral approach. It avoids the negotiation of the chopper below the capsulorhexis margin. Once the phaco probe is buried into the fragment, vacuum builts up. The peripheral chop is performed by pulling the nucleus out of the rhexis margin and then doing a chop **(Figure 16).** It is extremely useful in hard leathery cataracts.

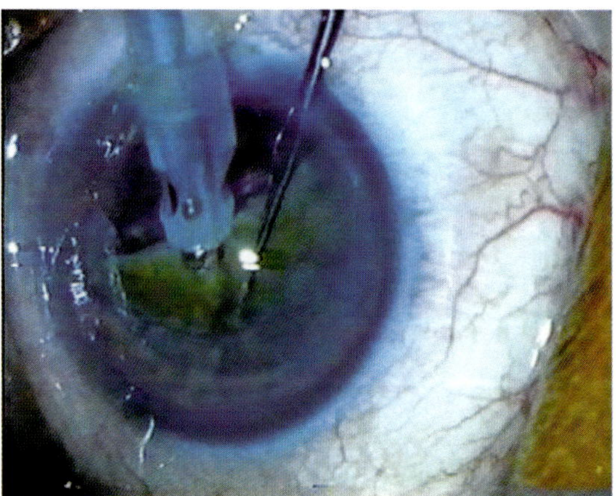

Figure 16: Modified peripheral chop with the nuclear fragment brought to the center.

REMOVAL OF NUCLEUS FRAGMENTS

Once each half of the nucleus is split into two or more fragments, each is held radially with a phacoprobe and moved centrally for its removal **(Figure 17)**.

The two systems of phaco machine—Peristaltic and Venturi behave differently. The peristaltic pump with low flow rate will have a weak attraction for the quadrant which can be increased moderately by increasing the flow rate while the venturi pump has a stronger attraction.

The phaco tip should be embedded in the quadrant using the phaco power, which is varied depending upon the density of the nucleus and the foot switch is then moved back to position 2. Occlusion allows the vacuum to build up and thus the nuclear fragment is moved centrally. Phaco power is used to remove the fragments, using the chopper in the other hand to divide nuclear fragment further or to feed it into the tip of the probe.

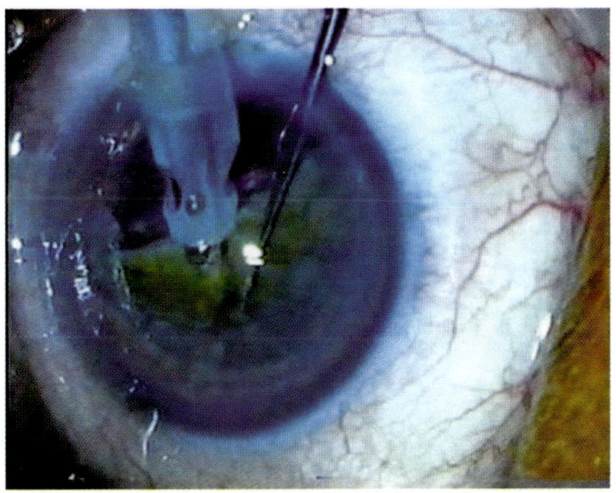

Figure 17: Each fragment is held radially and brought to center and emulsified.

Sometimes the continuous use of power may allow the probe to pass through and through the fragment, risking engaging the iris or capsule into the probe. In this case the surgeon should bring back the foot pedal to irrigation mode and position the fragment with the help of a second instrument through the side port and then proceed to emulsify it.

Subincisional Quadrant

The beginners may find it difficult to rotate a fragment at 12 o'clock position to 6 o'clock position. Viscoelastics is injected from the side port underneath the capsulorhexis margin at 12 o'clock position which pushes the fragment forward making it easy for the fragment to be engaged.

<u>Editorial Comment</u>

In order to achieve an efficient elimination of the nucleus by means of phacoemulsification, it is vital that the surgeon masters the different methods of using ultrasonic energy in the process: pulse mode, burst mode, hyperpulse mode, longitudinal and torsional ultrasound. All of the above methods, along with a command of different surgical techniques (e.g., Divide and Conquer, Stop and Chop, Flip and Chip, Direct Chop or Prechop), work together to make surgery safer to the corneal endothelium, the iris and the posterior capsule.

Arnaldo Espaillat, MD

Bibliography

1. Badoza D., Mendy JF, Ganly M. Phacoemulsification using the burst mode.J Cataract Refract Surg 2003; 29:1101-1105 © 2003.
2. Fine IH, Packer M, Hoffman RS. Power modulations in new phacoemulsification technology: improved outcomes. J Cataract Refract Surg 2004;30(5):1014-9.
3. Georgescu D, Payne M, Olson RJ. Objective measurement of postocclusion surge during phacoemulsification in human eye-bank eyes. Am J Ophthalmol. 2007;143(3):437-440.
4. Lal H, Sethi A. Manual of Phaco techniques. Text and Atlas.First edition. CBS Publishers 2002.
5. Mele B, Rosa. QuickChop Phacoemulsification: Technique and Tips. Techniques in Ophthalmology 2004 March;2(1):1-4.
6. Rekas M, Montés-Micó R, Krix-Jachym K, et al. Comparison of torsional and longitudinal modes using phacoemulsification parameters. J Cataract Refract Surg. 2009;35(10):1719-1724.
7. Seibel B.S. Mastering the Tools and Techniques of Phaco- emulsification Surgery, Third edition. Slack incorporated 1999;98.
8. Steinert RF. Phaco Chop. Ophthalmic surgery: Principles and Practice. (183-191) Philadelphia: WB Saunders, 2003.
9. Vasavada AR, Raj SM, Patel U, et al. Comparison of torsional and microburst longitudinal phacoemulsification: a prospective, randomized, masked clinical trial. Ophthalmic Surg Lasers Imaging. 2010;41(1):109-114.

5 | Transition from Standard Phacoemulsification to Bi-Manual Phaco

Amar Agarwal, MS
Athiya Agarwal, MD
Sunita Agarwal, MS

The problem with the small incision phaco technique (0.9 mm) was to find an IOL which would pass through such a small incision. Since 2001 the authors have gained extensive experience with the technique Phakonit (designed by Amar Agarwal) and the implantation of a Rollable IOL through a 0.9 mm size incision. This was done in their hospital at Chennai, India. The lens used was a special lens from ThinOptx. This lens used a Fresnel principle and was designed by Wayne Callahan from USA. The first such ultrathin lens was implanted by Dr. Jairo Hoyos from Spain. Dr. Amar Agarwal then modified this into a special 5 mm optic rollable IOL.

Principle

The problem in standard phacoemulsification is that we are not able to go below an incision of 3.0 mm. The reason is because of the infusion sleeve. The infusion sleeve takes up a lot of space. The titanium tip of the phaco handpiece has a diameter of 0.9 mm. This is surrounded by the infusion sleeve which allows fluid to pass into the eye. It also cools the handpiece tip so that a corneal burn does not occur.[3]

The authors separated the phaco tip from the infusion sleeve. In other words, the infusion sleeve was taken out. The tip was passed inside the eye and as there was no infusion sleeve present the size of the incision was smaller. In the left hand an irrigating chopper was held which had fluid passing inside the eye. The left hand was in the same position where the chopper is normally held; i.e.; the side port incision. The assistant applied fluid (BSS) continuously at the site of the incision to cool the phaco tip.

Terminology

The name PHAKONIT has been given because it shows phaco (PHAKO) being done with a needle (N) opening via an incision (I) and with the phako tip (T). This is also because it is Phako being done with a Needle Incision Technology. It is now internationally known as Bimanual phaco.

Transition to Bimanual Phaco

Anesthesia

The Bimanual Phaco Technique or Phakonit can be done under any type of anesthesia also. The authors have performed the procedure without any anesthetic drops.[4] The authors have analyzed that there is no difference between topical anesthesia cataract surgery and intracameral anesthesia cataract surgery. If the case is difficult one can use a peribulbar block.

Incision

In the first step a needle connected to a syringe with viscoelastic is pierced into the anterior chamber in the area where the side port has to be made. The viscoelastic is then injected into the eye. This will increase the IOP so that will be easier performing the clear corneal incision, which is done temporal. A special knife can be used for this purpose **(Figure 1)**. This keratome and other instruments for Phakonit are made by Huco (Switzerland) and Gueder (Germany).

Rhexis

The rhexis is done with a bent needle **(Figure 2)**. In the left hand a straight rod is held to stabilize the eye. The advantage of this is that the movements of the eye can get controlled.

Hydrodissection

Hydrodissection is performed and the fluid wave passing under the nucleus checked. Check for rotation of the nucleus. One should be careful when doing hydrodissection as there is not enough space for fluid to exit out.

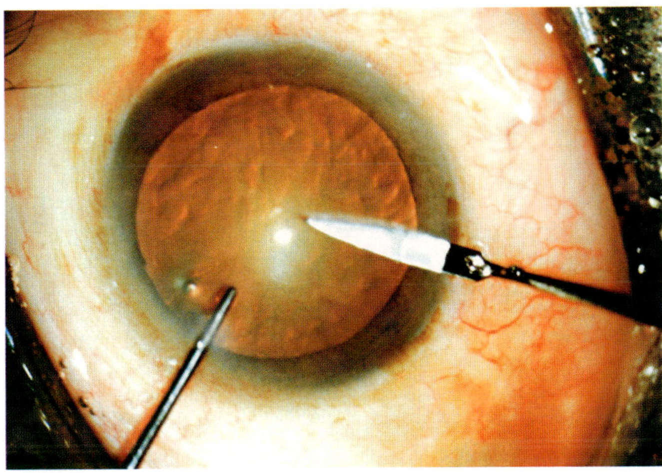

Figure 1: Clear corneal incision made with the keratome. Note the left hand has a straight rod to stabilize the eye as the case is done without any anesthesia. These instruments are made by Katena (USA).

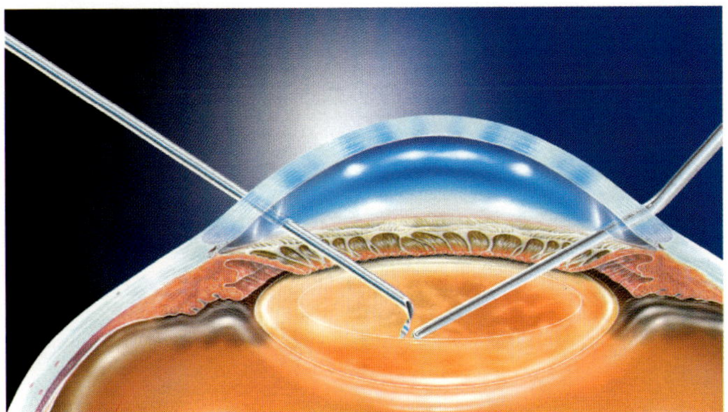

Figure 2: Rhexis started with a needle. (Art from Jaypee-Highligths).

Bimanual Phaco or Phakonit

Through the side port an irrigating chopper (Agarwal irrigating chopper) connected to the infusion line of the phaco machine is introduced with foot pedal on position 1. Other excellent irrigating choppers are David Chang's, Randall Olson's, Robert Osher's, Howard Fine's and Hiroshi Tsuneoka's irrigating chopper. Other choppers available are from Dr. F. Vejarano. The phaco probe is connected to the aspiration line and the phaco tip without an infusion sleeve is introduced through the clear corneal incision. Using the phaco tip with moderate ultrasound power, the center of the nucleus is directly embedded starting from the superior edge of rhexis with the phaco probe directed obliquely downwards towards the vitreous. The settings at this stage is 50% phaco power, flow rate 24 ml/min and 110 mm Hg vacuum. When nearly half of the center of nucleus is embedded, the foot pedal is moved to position 2 as it helps to hold the nucleus due to vacuum rise. To avoid undue pressure on the posterior capsule, the nucleus is lifted slightly and the nucleus is chopped with the irrigating chopper in the left hand. This is done with a straight downward motion from the inner edge of the rhexis to the center of the nucleus and then to the left in the shape of an inverted L **(Figure 3)**. Once the crack is created, the nucleus is split till the center. The nucleus is then rotated 180º and cracked again so that the nucleus is completely split into two halves.

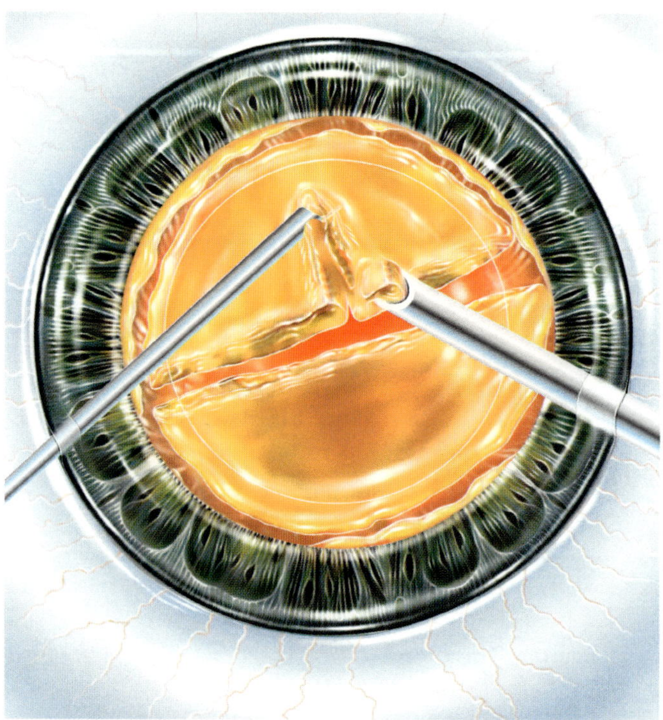

Figure 3: Phakonit started. Note the phako needle in the right hand and an irrigating chopper in the left hand. Phakonit being performed. Note the crack created by karate chopping. The assistant continuously irrigates the phaco probe area from outside to prevent corneal burns. (Art from Jaypee-Highligths).

The nucleus is then rotated 90º and embedding done in one half of the nucleus with the probe directed horizontally. With the previously described technique, 3 pie-shaped fragments are created in each half of the nucleus. With a short burst of energy at pulse mode, each pie shaped fragment is lifted and brought at the level of iris where it is further emulsified and aspirated sequentially in pulse mode. Thus the whole nucleus is removed **(Figure 4)**. Cortical wash-up is done with the bimanual irrigation aspiration technique **(Figure 5)**.

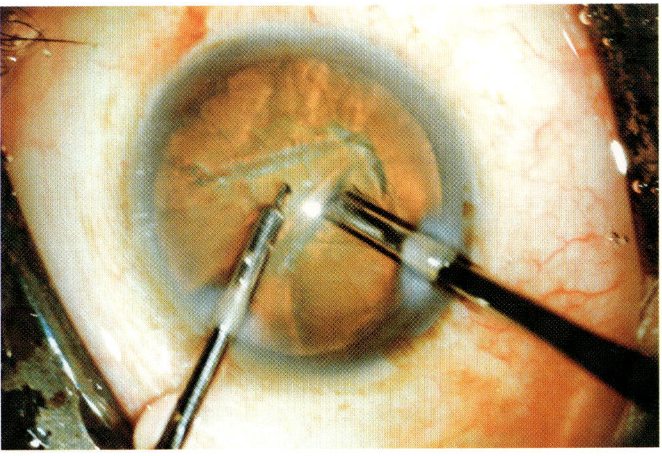

Figure 4: Phakonit completed. Note the nucleus has been removed and there are no corneal burns.

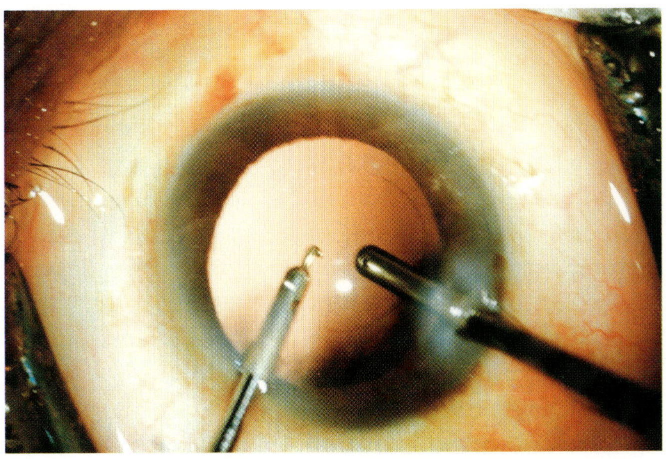

Figure 5: Bimanual irrigation aspiration completed.

AC Stability in Phakonit

The main problem in Phakonit is that the amount of fluid entering the eye through the irrigating chopper is less than the amount of fluid exiting the eye through the sleeveless phaco needle.

Diferent surgeons have tried different methods to solve this problem of anterior chamber stability. The various methods are:
1. Air Pump or Anti-chamber collapser[5]
2. Anterior Vented Gas Forced Infusion System (VGFI) of the Accurus Surgical System
3. STAAR Surgical's disposable Cruise Control device
4. Well designed Irrigating choppers.

Air Pump

One of the limitations in bimanual phaco is the destabilization of anterior chamber during surgery. This has been overcome by the introduction of gas forced infusion by Dr. Sunita Agarwal.[5] Another development made by us (SA) was to use an air pump or anti-chamber collapser which injects air into the infusion bottle **(Figure 6)**. This pushes in more fluid into the eye through the irrigating chopper and also prevents surge. Thus we were not only able to use a 20 gauge irrigating chopper but also solve the problem of destabilization of the anterior chamber during surgery. This increases the steady-state pressure of the eye making the anterior chamber deep and well maintained during the entire procedure. It even makes phacoemulsification a relatively safe procedure by reducing surge even at high vacuum levels. Thus this can be used not only in Phakonit but also in Phacoemulsification.[6]

Surge

When a fragment occluding the tip is held by high vacuum, and then abruptly aspirated, fluid rushes into the phaco tip to equilibrate the built up vacuum in the aspiration line, causing surge. This leads to shallowing or collapse of the anterior chamber. Different machines employ a variety of methods to combat surge. These include usage of noncomplaint tubing[7], small bore aspiration line tubing[7], microflow tips[7], aspiration bypass systems[7], dual linear foot pedal control[7] and incorporation of sophisticated microprocessors[7] to sense the anterior chamber pressure fluctuations.

The surgeon dependent variables to counteract surge include good wound construction with minimal leakage[8] and selection of appropriate machine parameters depending on the stage of the surgery.[8] An anterior chamber maintainer

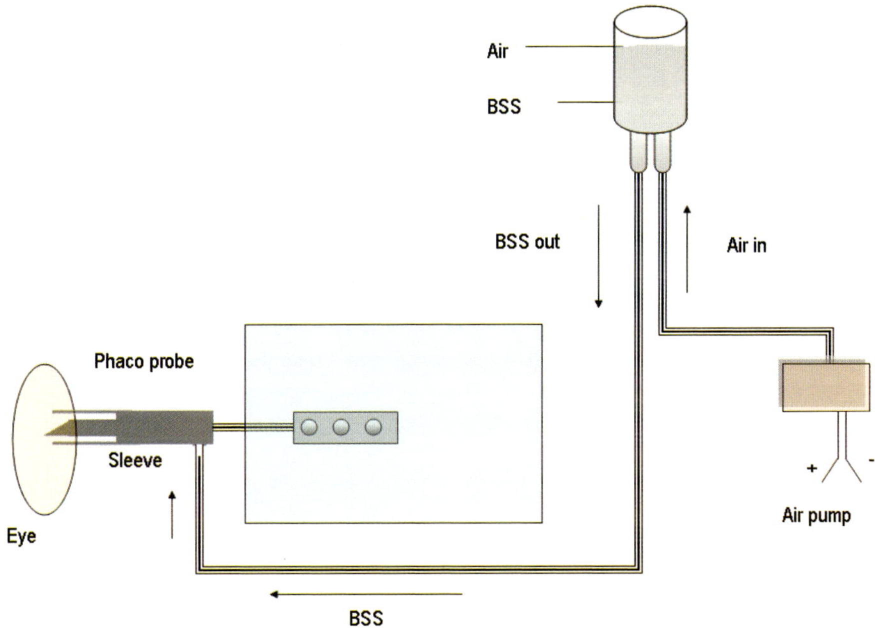

Figure 6: Anti-chamber collapser.

has also been described in literature to prevent surge, but an extra side port makes it an inconvenient procedure. Another method to solve surge is to use more of phacoaspiration and chop the nucleus into smaller pieces.

Technique

An IV set is used to connect the BSS bottle to the irrigation tubing of the handpiece **(Figure 6)**. The bottles are kept at a height of about 65 centimeters above the operating field. The automated air pump, which is similar to the pump used in aquariums to supply oxygen to the fish, is utilized to forcefully pump air into the irrigation bottle at a continuous rate.

With this increased fluid volume we were able to maintain a deep anterior chamber and no surge was observed in our routine Phakonit or phacoemulsification cases.

Discussion

Surge is caused by the volume of the fluid forced out of the eye into the aspiration line at the instant of occlusion break. When the phacoemulsification handpiece tip is occluded, flow is interrupted and vacuum builds up to its maximal preset values. Additionally the aspiration tubing may collapse in the presence of high vacuum levels. Emulsification of the occluding fragment clears the block and the fluid rushes into the aspiration line to neutralize the pressure difference created between the positive pressure in the anterior chamber and the negative pressure in the aspiration tubing. In addition, if the aspiration line tubing is not reinforced to prevent collapse (tubing compliance), the tubing, constricted during occlusion, then expands on occlusion break. These factors cause a rush of fluid from the anterior chamber into the phaco probe. The fluid in the anterior chamber is not replaced rapidly enough to prevent shallowing of the anterior chamber.

The maintenance of intra ocular pressure (steady–state IOP) during the entire procedure depends on the equilibrium between the fluid inflow and outflow. In most phacoemulsification machines, fluid inflow is provided by gravitational flow of the fluid from the balanced salt solution (BSS) bottle through the tubing to the anterior chamber. This is determined by the bottle height relative to the patient's eye, the diameter of the tubing and most importantly by the outflow of fluid from the eye through the aspiration tube and leakage from the wounds.

The inflow volume can be increased by either rising the bottle height or by enlarging the diameter of the inflow tube. The intraocular pressure augments by 10 mm Hg for every 15 centimeters increment in bottle height above the eye.[7] High steady-state IOPs increase phaco safety by raising the mean IOP level up and away from zero, i.e. by delaying surge related anterior chamber collapse. Air pump increases the amount of fluid inflow thus making the steady-state IOP high. This deepens the anterior chamber, increasing the surgical space available for maneuvering and thus prevents complications like posterior capsular tears and corneal endothelial damage. The phenomenon of surge is neutralized by rapid inflow of fluid at the time of occlusion break. The recovery to steady-state IOP is so prompt that no surge occurs and this enables the surgeon to remain in foot position 3 through the occlusion break. High vacuum phacoemulsification can be safely performed in hard brown cataracts using an air pump. Phacoemulsification under topical or no anesthesia[9] can be safely done neutralizing the positive vitreous pressure occurring due to squeezing of the eyelids.

Anterior Vented Gas Forced Infusion System (AVGFI) of the Accurus Surgical System (ALCON)

This was started by Arturo Pérez-Arteaga, MD from Mexico. The AVGFI is a system incorporated in the Accurus machine that creates a positive infusion pressure inside the eye; it was designed by the Alcon engineers to control the intraocular pressure (IOP) during the anterior and posterior segment surgery. It consist of an air pump and a regulator which are inside the machine; then the air is pushed inside the bottle of intraocular solution, and so the fluid is actively pushed inside the eye without raising the bottle. The control of the air pump is digitally integrated in the Accurus panel; it also can be controlled via the remote. Also the footswitch can be preset with the minimum and maximum of desired inflow to the eye and go directly to this values with the simple touch of the footswitch. Arturo Pérez-Arteaga recommends to preset the infusion pump at 100 to 110 cm H_2O; it is enough strong irrigation force to perform a microincision phaco. This parameter is preset in the panel and also as the minimal irrigation force in the footswitch; then he recommends to preset the maximal irrigation force at 130 to 140 cm H_2O in the foot pedal, so if a surge exist during the procedure the surgeon can increase the irrigation force by the simple touch of the footswitch to the right. With the AVGFI the surgeon has the capability to increase even more these values.

Cruise Control (STAAR Surgical)

The Cruise Control is a disposable, flow-restricting (0.3-mm internal diameter) device that is placed in between the phaco handpiece and the aspiration tubing of any phaco machine. The goal is very similar to that of the flare tip (Alcon): combining a standard phaco tip opening with a narrower shaft to provide more grip with less surge. This has been popularized by David Chang, MD (USA) for phakonit surgery. STAAR Surgical introduced this disposable Cruise Control device, which can be used with any phaco machine.

Duet System

Larry Laks (USA) created the Duet system (Microsurgical Technology-MST). The advantage of this is that it is a whole bimanual phaco set for Phakonit. The Duet system has Phakonit knives also **(Figure 7)** and also handles on which various irrigating choppers can fit **(Figure 8)**. The   Microsurgical

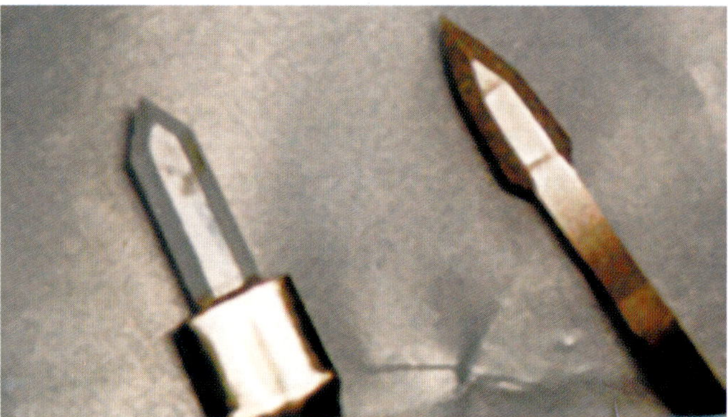

Figure 7: Phakonit knives. The one on the left is the Agarwal sapphire phakonit knife made by Huco (Switzerland). The one on the right is the one made by Microsurgical Technology.

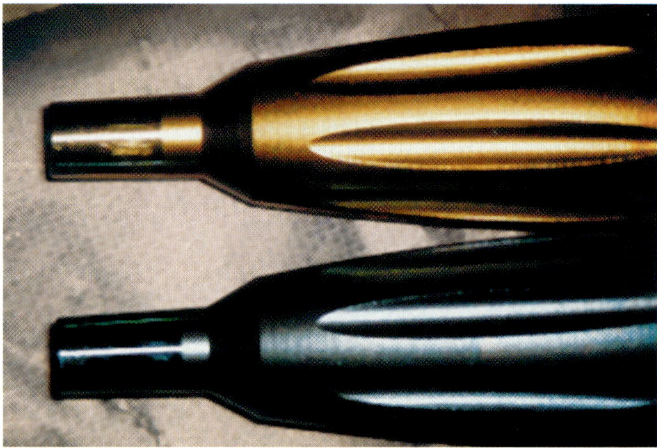

Figure 8: Duet system. These are the handles of the Duet system (Microsurgical Technology). The irrigating choppers and bimanual irrigation aspiration sets can be interchanged with the handles.

Technologies (MST) 20-gauge Duet irrigating choppers provide the best inflow of comparable devices. The MST shaft design gives an impressive inflow rate of 40 cc/min at 30 in of bottle height and is available with an assortment of interchangeable chopper tips. The idea was to have the opening in the irrigating choppers larger. The clear corneal incision can be created with the MST knife **(Figure 9)** and then Phakonit started using the Agarwal sharp MST irrigating chopper **(Figure 10)**. Once Phakonit is completed the Bimanual Irrigation aspiration set from the Duet system is used and the cortical aspiration completed.

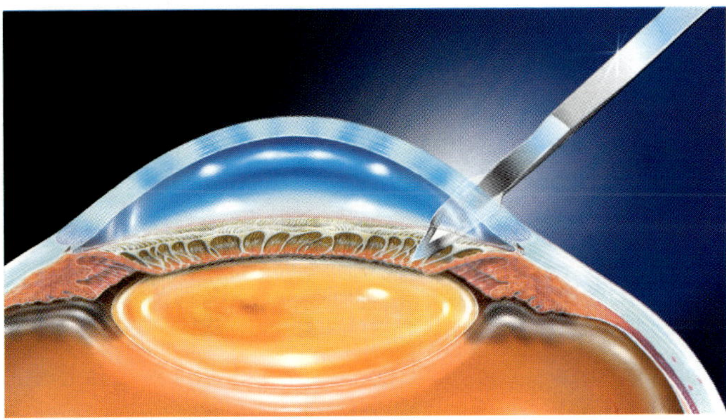

Figure 9: Clear corneal incision made with the Microsurgical Technology knife. (Art from Jaypee-Highligths).

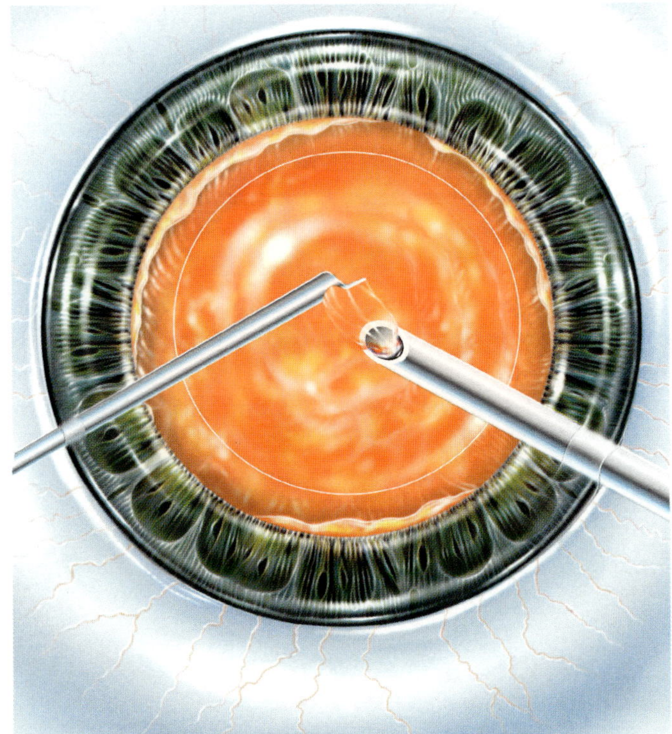

Figure 10: Phakonit being done with the Agarwal sharp irrigating chopper from Microsurgical Technology. (Art from Jaypee-Highligths).

ThinOptx Rollable IOL

ThinOptx, the company that manufactures these lenses has a patented technology that allows the manufacture of lenses with plus or minus 30 diopters of correction on the thickness of 100 microns. The ThinOptx technology is not limited to material choice, but instead is achieved by a revolutionary optic and unprecedented nano-scale manufacturing process. The lens is made from off-the-shelf hydrophilic material, which is similar to several IOL materials already on the market. The key to the ThinOptx lens is the optic design and nano-precision manufacturing. The basic advantage of this lens is that they are ultra-thin lenses.

Lens Insertion Technique

The lens is held with a forceps **(Figure 11)**. The lens is then placed in a bowl of BSS solution that is approximately body temperature. This makes the lens pliable. Once the lens is pliable it is taken with the gloved hand holding it between the index finger and the thumb. The lens is then rolled in a rubbing motion. It is preferable to do this in the bowl of BSS so that the lens remains rolled well.

Note: Several injectors have been developed for the ThinOptx. The group of Dr. L. Felipe Vejarano from Colombia have found very useful the last generation one, which consists of two pieces. One is a cartridge (roller head) that features a slot, and is attached to a syringe, and a second piece (button) with a plate in the forward portion, which fits into the slot of the cartridge. The "button" has a rounded rear portion to make easier to press on it using the thumb, and acts as a plunger to push the IOL deep into the slot. The surgeon must keep the "button" pressed for 5 seconds, before injecting the IOL **(Figure 12)**.

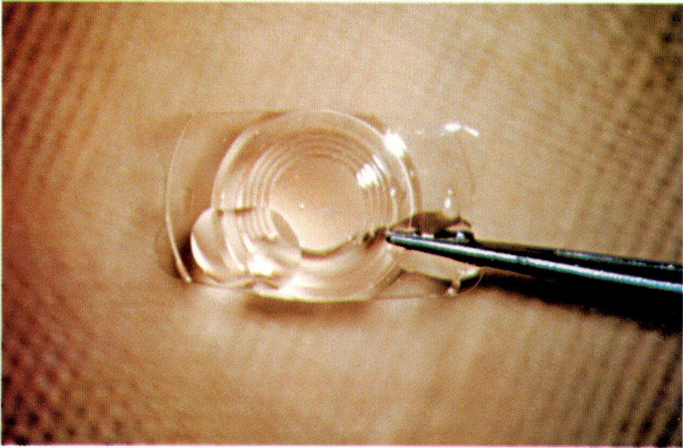

Figure 11: The phakonit ThinOptx rollable IOL when removed from the bottle.

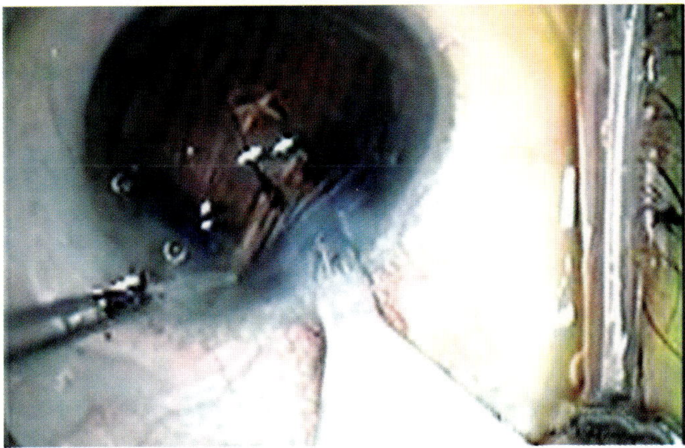

Figure 12: While holding the eye with a second instrument through the side port incision, the leading haptic of the IOL is implanted inside the bag. (Courtesy of Dr. L. Felipe Vejarano- Colombia).

The lens is then inserted through the sub 1.4 mm incision carefully. One can then move the lens into the capsular bag. The natural warmth of the eye causes the lens to open gradually. Viscoelastic is then removed with the Bimanual irrigation aspiration probes **(Figure 13)**. The tips of the footplates are extremely thin which allow the lens to be positioned with the footplates rolled to fit the bag.

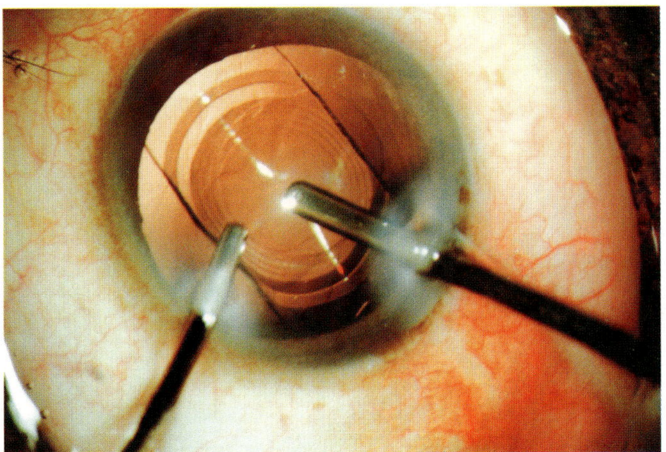

Figure 13: Viscoelastic removed using bimanual irrigation aspiration probes.

Topography

We perfomed topography with the Orbscan™ to compare cases of phakonit and standard phaco and we found that the induced astigmatism in phakonit cases is much lower **(Figures 14, 15)**. Stabilization of refraction is also faster with Phakonit compared to phaco surgery.

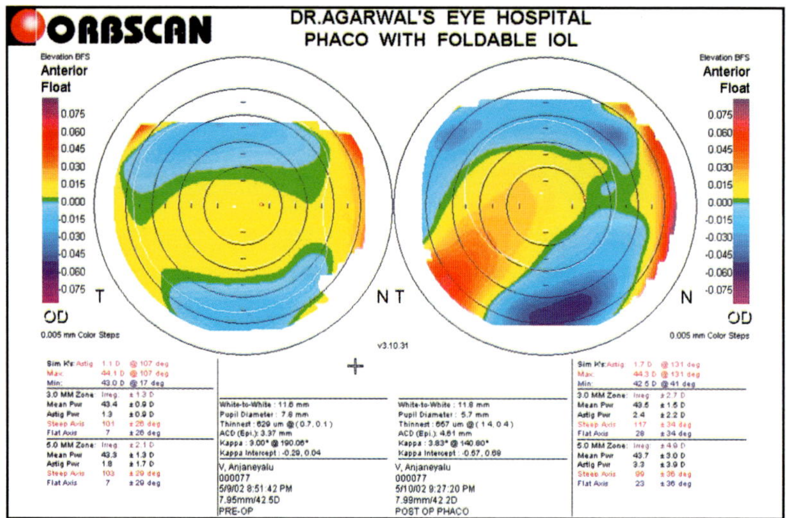

Figure 14: Phako foldable IOL Orbscan™ results. Left: pre-operative exam. Right: one day post-operative exam. Note the difference between the two topography pictures. This is the site where the clear corneal temporal incision was made.

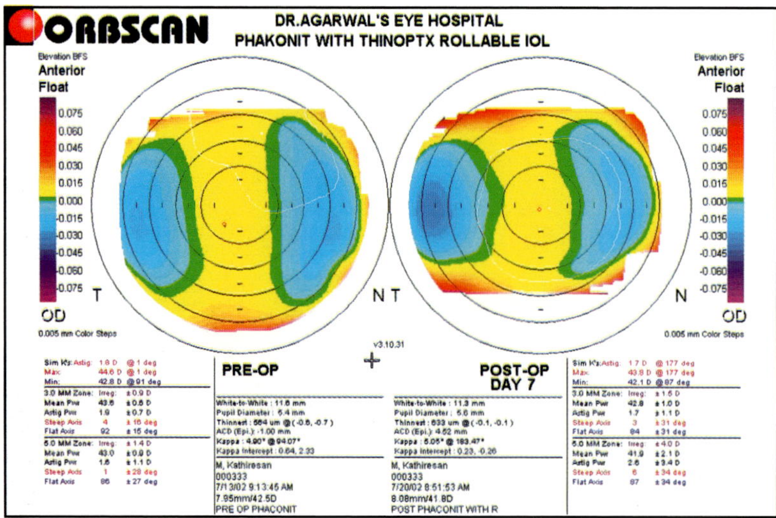

Figure 15: Phakonit with a rollable IOL Orbscan™ results.

Acri.Tec IOL

The Acry.Lye IOL is manufactured by the Acri.Tec company in Berlin, Germany. The intraocular lens **(Figure 16)** consists of highly purified biocompatible hydrophobic acrylate with chemically bonded UV-absorber. It is a single piece foldable IOL like a plate-haptic IOL. The lens is sterilized by autoclaving. The lens comes in a sterile vial, filled with water and wrapped in a sterile pouch.

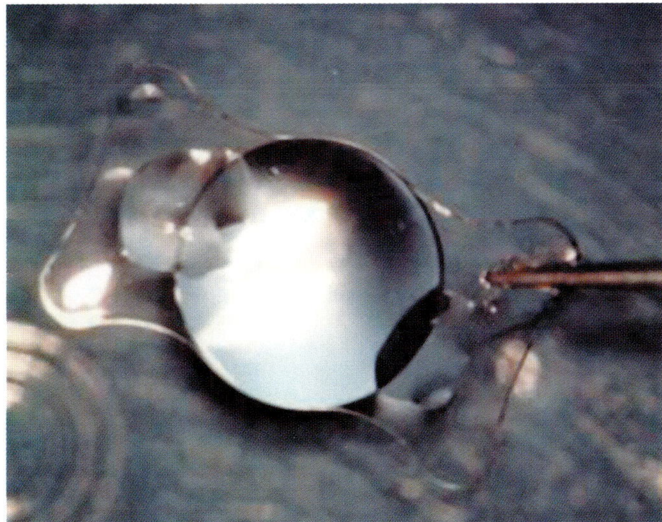

Figure 16: The Acri.Lye foldable IOL.

Lens Loading and Insertion Technique

After the Phakonit procedure is completed, the incision is increased to 1.5 mm. The lens is like a plate haptic IOL. It is implanted using an injector. First of all the injector tip is fitted with a sponge tip which comes with the cartridge. This will prevent the injector tip from damaging the lens while inserting it inside the eye. The lens is then taken out from the bottle /vial, held with a forceps, and placed in the cartridge. Viscoelastic is injected in the cartridge and once the flanges of the IOL are in the groove of the cartridge, it is closed and then inserted in the injector. Once the cartridge is fixed onto the injector, the plunger is pressed making the sponge tip to push the lens till one can see it coming into the nozzle of the cartridge **(Figure 17)**. The inferior haptic goes into the bag and the superior haptic is gradually tucked inside the capsular bag **(Figure 18)**.

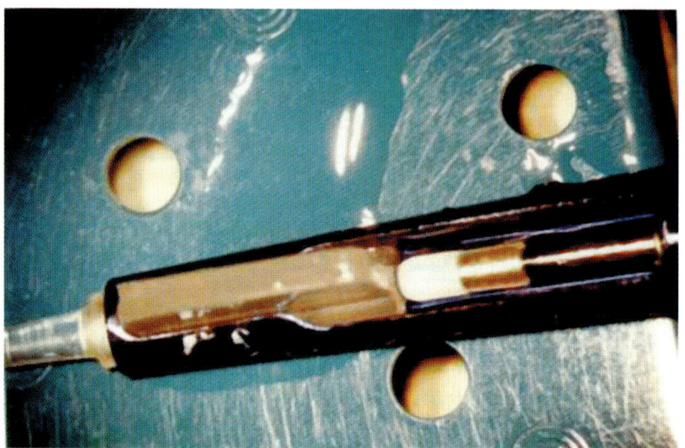

Figure 17: The tip of the Acri.Tec injector with the sponge tip ready in place to push the IOL.

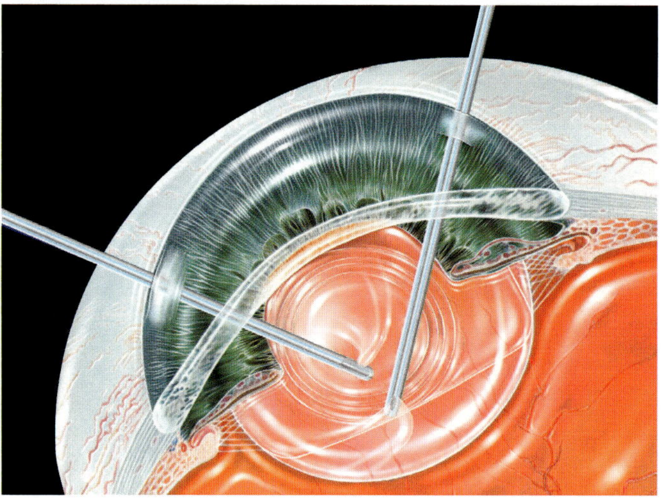

Figure 18: Viscoelastic removed using bimanual irrigation aspiration probes.

Summary

There are various problems, which are encountered in any innovative technique and so also with Phakonit, but with time these will have to be solved. The important point is that even today we have broken the 1 mm barrier for cataract removal. This can be done easily by separating the phaco needle from the infusion sleeve. As the saying goes- "We have miles to go before we can sleep". The differences between Phaco and Phakonit are shown in **Table 1**.

Table 1 : Difference Between Phako and Phakonit.

PHAKO vs. PHAKONIT

FEATURE	PHAKO	PHAKONIT
1.INCISION SIZE	3 MM	SUB 1.4 MM
2.AIR PUMP	NOT MANDATORY	MANDATORY
3. HAND USAGE	SINGLE HANDED PHACO POSSIBLE	TWO HANDS (BIMANUAL)
4.NON DOMINANT HAND ENTRY AND EXIT	LAST TO ENTER AND FIRST TO EXIT	FIRST TO ENTER AND LAST TO EXIT
5.CAPSULORHEXIS	NEEDLE OR FORCEPS	BETTER WITH NEEDLE
6.IOL	FOLDABLE IOL	ROLLABLE IOL
7.ASTIGMATISM	TWO UNEQUAL INCISIONS CREATE ASTIGMATISM	TWO EQUAL ULTRASMALL INCISIONS NEGATE THE INDUCED ASTIGMATISM
8.STABILITY OF REFRACTION	LATER THAN PHAKONIT	EARLIER THAN PHACO
9.IRIS PROLAPSE-INTRAOPERATIVE	MORE CHANCES	LESS CHANCES DUE TO SMALLER INCISION

References

1. Sunita Agarwal, Athiya Agarwal, Mahipal S Sachdev, Keiki R Mehta, I Howard Fine, Amar Agarwal: Phaco emulsification, Laser Cataract Surgery & Foldable IOL's;Second edition Jaypee Brothers; 2000, Delhi, India
2. Benjamin F Boyd, Sunita Agarwal, Athiya Agarwal, Amar Agarwal: Lasik and Beyond Lasik; Highlights of Ophthalmology; 2000, Panama
3. Laura J Ronge: Clinical Update; Five Ways to avoid Phaco Burns; February 1999
4. Agarwal A, Jacob S, Sinha S, Agarwal A.Combating endophthalmitis with microphakonit and no-anesthesia technique. J Cataract Refract Surg. 2007 Dec;33(12):2009-11
5. Agarwal A, Agarwal S, Agarwal A, Lal V, Patel N. Antichamber collapser.J Cataract Refract Surg. 2002 Jul;28(7):1085-6
6. Chaudhry P, Prakash G, Jacob S, Narasimhan S, Agarwal S, Agarwal A. Safety and efficacy of gas-forced infusion (air pump) in coaxial phacoemulsification. J Cataract Refract Surg. 2010 Dec;36(12):2139-45
7. Fishkind WJ. The Phaco Machine : How and why it acts and reacts? In: Agarwal's Four volume textbook of Ophthalmology. Jaypee Brothers: New Delhi; 2000.
8. Seibel SB. The fluidics and physics of phaco. In: Agarwal's et al. Phacoemulsification, Laser cataract surgery and foldable IOLs Second edition. Jaypee Brothers: New Delhi; 2000; 45-54.
9. Agarwal et al. No anesthesia cataract surgery with karate chop; In: Agarwal's Phacoemulsification, Laser cataract surgery and foldable IOLs Second Edition Second Edition. Jaypee Brothers: New Delhi; 2000; 217-226.

6 | Micro-Incision Cataract Surgery (MICS)

Jorge L. Alio, MD, PhD
Jose-Luis Rodriguez Prats, MD
Ahmed Galal MD, PhD

The Trends Towards Microincision Cataract Surgery (MICS)

Biaxial microincision clear corneal phacoemulsification was created as a an innovative method which made the corneal incision smaller. This method was described by Shearing in 1985.[1] This procedure uses separate irrigations with an irrigating chopper, sleeveless phacoemulsification tip, and also requires pulsed phacoemulsification energy.

The minimization of the incision is a consequence of a natural evolution of the cataract surgery technique in the search of excellence. When we place cataract surgery within the context of Gaussian distribution, it is clear that the standard of practice today is through coaxial phacoemulsification **(Figure 1)**. Extracapsular 6 mm surgery is a procedure still in practice today, but less performed every

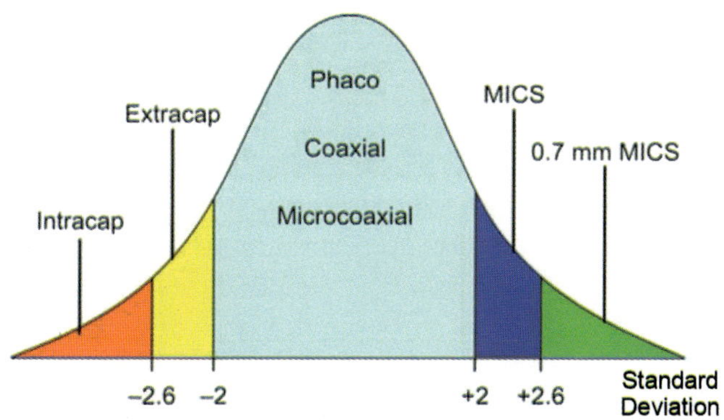

Figure 1: Natural evolution of cataract surgery.

day, hence between -2 and -2.6 standard deviation. The Gaussian curve is like a wave. It moves from ancient to new surgical techniques. Nowadays the standard coaxial technique is still the most popular type of cataract surgery in the world. The coaxial wound size is still 2.75 mm, in spite of the availability of the newest foldable intraocular lenses which can be injected through smaller incisions. Microincision Cataract Surgery (MICS) can make the incision smaller than 1.5 mm and it should be considered beyond the 2 up to the 2.6 standard deviations of our Gaussian distribution. MICS will be the standard of practice in future, and what we could call sub 1 mm MICS or micro-MICS will be the next standard.[2] MICS is the next stage in the evolution of cataract surgery.

Required Elements for MICS

Fluidics optimization: Basically MICS means operating in a closed chamber. It is necessary to optimize the balance between the outflow and inflow, determined by the flow rate of the irrigating instruments, a function of its diameter and the fluid pressure; the volume of fluid aspirated throught the tip; and the amount of leakage through the incisions.[3]

Bimanuality and separation of functions: Means working with irrigation and aspiration as separated instruments in both hands of the surgeon.[3]

New micro-instruments: Micro-instruments have been designed to perform specific functions in addition of providing inflow at the same time, which plays a crucial role in the fluidics balance. With the new maneuvers the efficiency of phacoemulsification is increased.[3]

Lasers: The very low levels of energy delivered into the eye when using laser in MICS and the possibilities of improving the efficiency of this technology in the future, make laser MICS surgery an attractive alternative.

Ultrasonic probes: New ultrasonic probes are designed to be more efficient and manipuled through micro-incisions without excessively stretching the corneal tissue. Furthermore, they have special protections or a smooth external surface to diminish friction between the probe and the tissue.

Indication for MICS Surgery

There is no limitation to indicate a MICS cataract operation. You can operate all grades of cataract LOCS III, even hard cataracts. The subluxated lenses, posttraumatic lenses, zonular laxity and congenital cataracts can also be operated with MICS, with small doses of ultrasound. Generally MICS does not induce astigmatism. MICS is especially dedicated for "refractive cataract operation". MICS can be used for refractive cataract surgery by injecting multifocal lenses and toric lenses.[4,5]

MICS Technique Advantages

Performing micro incision in cataract surgery has a number of theoretical advantages:

- Fast visual recovery and improved visual outcome.
- Decrease in induced astigmatism.
- Reduction in the healing time.
- Less complications.
- IOL insertion through microincision.

The emulsification of all grades of nucleus density could be achieved by improving the safety and the fluidics of the low US phaco and laser, with the possibility of managing greater aspiration and vacuum, and for the laser, maintaining continuous contact between the crystalline material and the laser aperture **(Table 1)**.

Table 1: Low Ultrasound MICS. Operative Parameters of the Phacoemulsificator Machine

A. Phaco parameters
Aspiration: 550 cc/min
Energy: 70 (20% - 30%) Joules
Flow rate: 20 cc/min
B. MICS operative parameters
Aspiration: 550 cc/min
Energy: 30 Joules
Flow rate: 20 cc/min

Surgical Instruments used in MICS Surgery

1) MICS Micro blade: is a diamond or stainless steel blade that is able to create a trapezoidal incision from 1.2 to 1.4-mm **(Figure 2A-B)**.[6]

2) MICS capsulorhexis forceps: It has micro triangular tips that can be used to puncture and grasp the capsule to perform the capsulorrhexis with a single instrument **(Figure 3)**.[7]

3) MICS Pre-choppers: they are to be used bimanually in all types of cataracts regardless of the hardness. The tip has a blunted square hook that should be introduced gently underneath the anterior capsular rim, one instrument opposite to the other.[6]

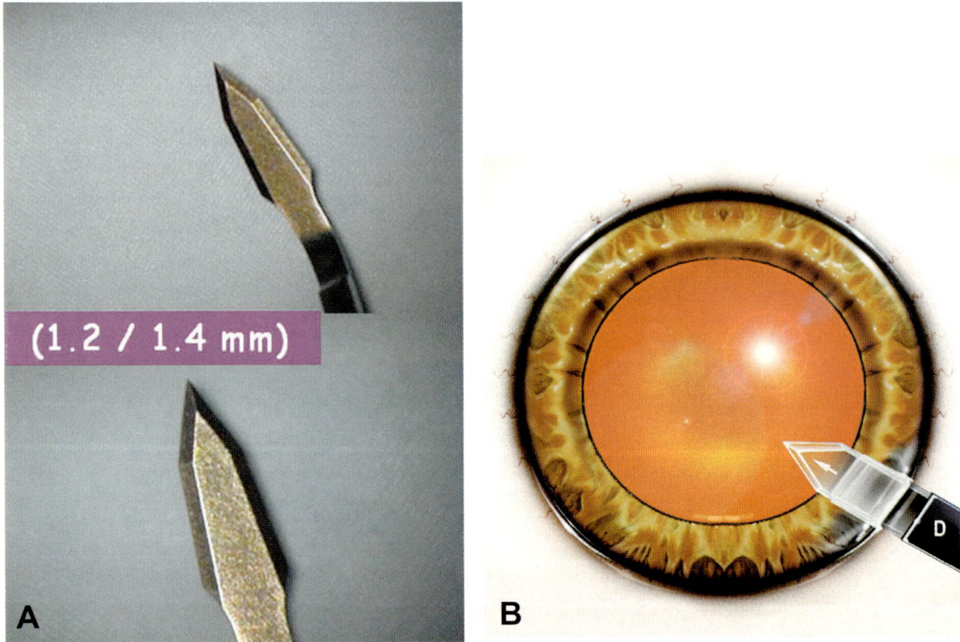

Figure 2 A-B: Alio's MICS microblade. (Figure 2B: Art from Jaypee Highlights).

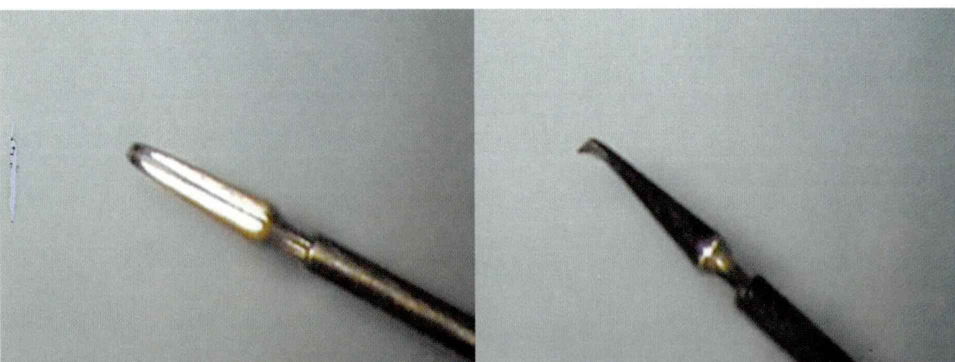

Figure 3: Alio's MICS Capsulorhexis forceps.

4) MICS hydrodissector or irrigating-Fingernail: capable of manipulating nucleus fragments as easy as the irrigating instrument. This can also be useful to further divide the nuclear fragments. The flow rate or the free irrigation flow of this onstrument is 72 cc/min that catenates anterior chamber stability regardless of the level of the high vacuum in MICS **(Figure 4)**.[7]

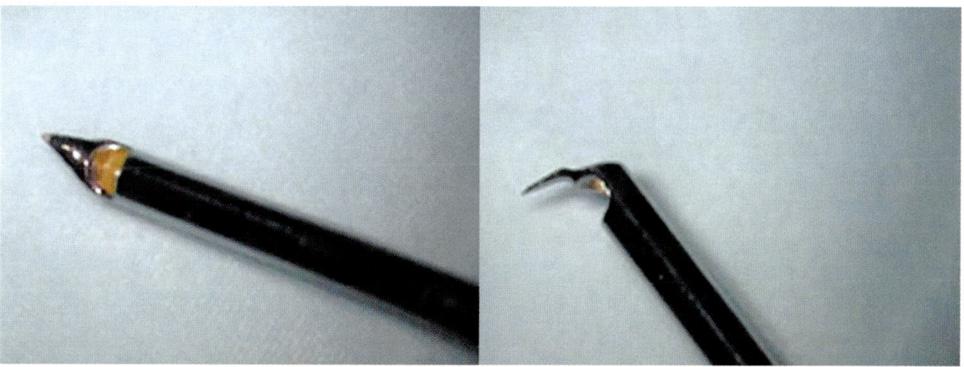

Figure 4: Alio's MICS hydromanipulator irrigating fingernail.

5) MICS irrigating Chopper: This instrument was designed to chop medium to hard cataract if pre-chopping has not been performed. It has a sharp pointed triangular shaped tip, which is angled downward to "chop" off segments of the nucleus **(Figure 5)**.[8]

6) MICS aspiration handpiece: The bullet shaped tip is designed for easy entry through a paracentesis incision and has a 0.3-mm diameter aspirating port close to the tip in the interior part of the curvature.

7) Intraocular Manipulator: The manipulator is multifunctional and efficiently helps in iridolenticular synechia dissection, IOL manipulation and other intraocular maneuvers such as vitreous strands or stabilization of the IOL. The conical base is the same diameter as the internal MICS incision in order to keep the anterior chamber stability thus preventing viscoelastic outflow.[8]

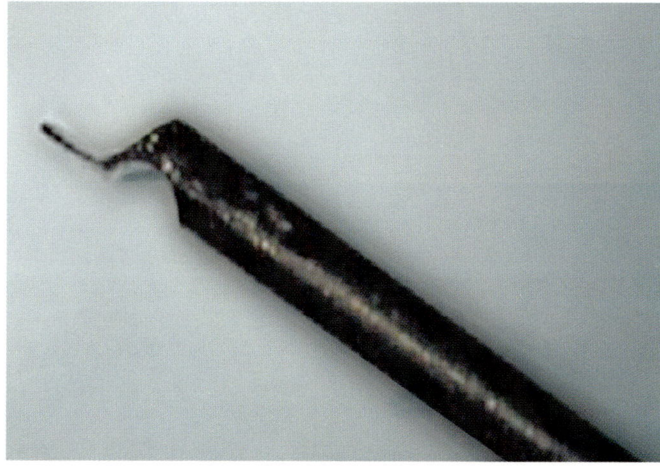

Figure 5: Alio's MICS irrigating chopper.

8) MICS scissors: The design is 23 gauge (0.6-mm) shaft, making it fit through a very small paracentesis. It has extremely delicate blunt tipped blades, which are ideal for cutting synechia and capsular fibrosis and membranes as well as for performing small iridotomies.

Low Ultrasound (LUS) –MICS Surgical Principles

The MICS technique can be performed using phacoemulsification, which is termed low ultrasound MICS (LUS-MICS), and by using laser which is termed laser-MICS. After termination of pre-chopping the Accurus™ or the Infiniti™ machines are adjusted according to the previous described settings.

Incisions

After the surgical field is isolated and an adjustable eye speculum is inserted, the steeper corneal meridian is marked and 2 trapezoidal incisions of 1.2 mm internally and 1.4 mm externally are performed using the Alio's corneal keratome **(Figure 6)**. With this, an external incision of 1.4 mm will be adequate for better instrument manipulation. The two incisions are performed in clear cornea 90º apart, at 10 and 2 o'clock **(Figure 7)** followed by the injection of 1% Lidocaine preservative free diluted 1:1 in BSS.

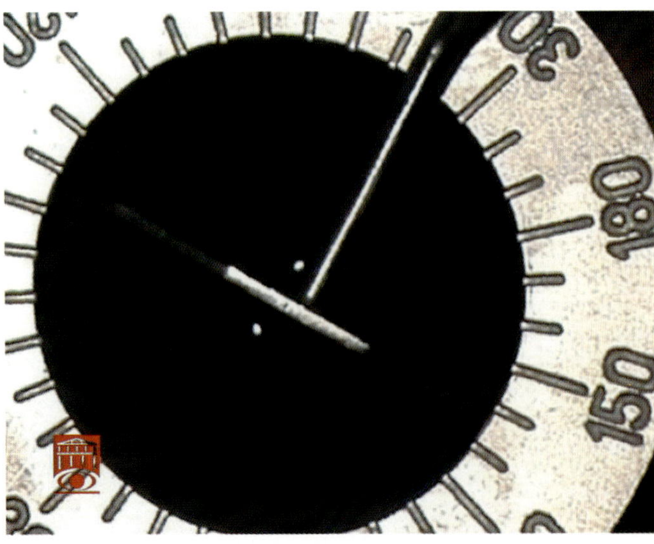

Figure 6: Marking of the corneal main incision at the steeper corneal meridian.

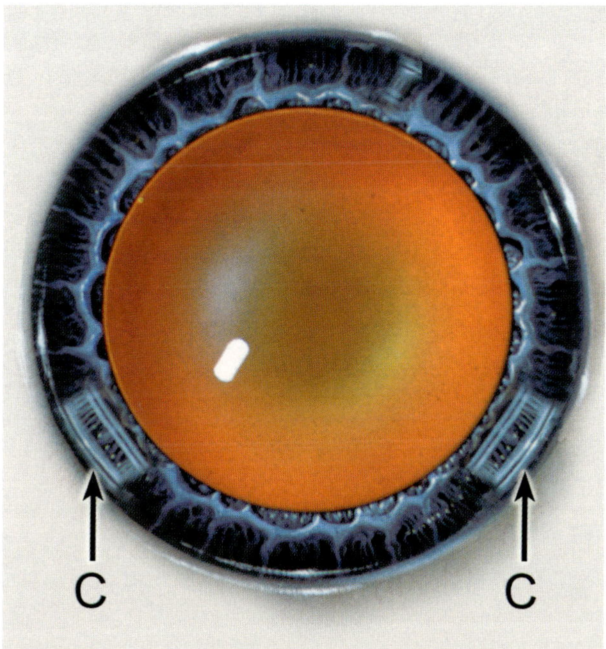

Figure 7: MICS 2 clear corneal incisions performed 90° apart (C). (Art from Jaypee Highlights).

Pre-chopping (Counter Chopping Technique)

After performing the capsulorhexis using Alio's capsulorhexis forceps, the prechopping is performed **(Figure 8).** This is a bimanual technique requiring the use of both hands with the same efficiency. This technique allows manual cut division of the nucleus, without creating any grooves prior to the MICS procedure. In order to protect the endothelium and to perform an adequate counter chopping technique, more dispersive or cohesive viscoelastic material is injected. The technique of counter prechopping could be applied to all surgical grades of cataract density (up to grade +5). A chopper is introduced through one of the 2 incisions depending on the surgeon's preference. Through the other incision a nuclear manipulator is introduced to decrease the stress on the capsule and zonules being inserted beneath the anterior capsulorhexis edge and the rounded microball tip of the nuclear manipulator will protect the posterior capsule during the prechopping procedure. The tips of the nuclear manipulator and the chopper should be aligned on the same axis together with the hardest point of the nucleus along the direction of the lens fibers then appropriate force is applied between the two instruments **(Figure 9).** After cracking the nucleus into fragments, the nucleus is rotated and the maneuver is repeated on the other axis to crack the nucleus into 4 quadrants.

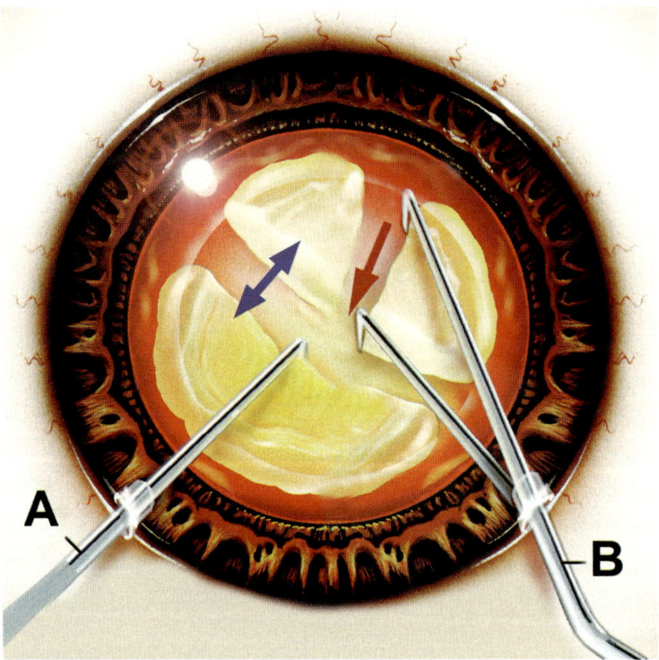

Figure 8: Pre-chopping maneuver manual cut division of the nucleus. (Art from Jaypee Highlights).

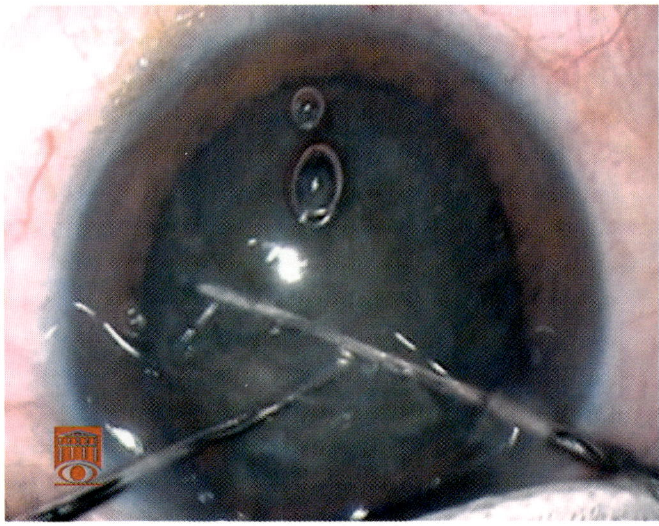

Figure 9: Pre-chopping.

In the case of soft cataracts having established the pressure at 500-550 mm Hg we can only use Alio's MICS hydromanipulator irrigating fingernail. This makes it possible to divide and aspirate fragments of the cataract without using ultrasound or using ultrasound in the minimum way. In this case, a torsional phacoemulsification system can be helpful. In the case of hard cataracts, when total occlusion of the tip occurs preventing aspiration, Alio's MICS Irrigating Stinger would be more useful. This handpiece has a narrow edge at the end which divides the masses and allows easy aspiration of the phacoemulsification tip. The fragmented elements of the hard cataracts are now easily aspirated using the high under pressure and in occasionally using ultrasound energy.

Using this technique reduces the tendency for the nuclear material to come up into the anterior chamber during the procedure maintaining its position within the epinuclear cover **(Figure 10)**. Following the emulsification of all the nuclear segments, the epinuclear rim is trimmed in the different quadrants in such way to remove all the cortical material remaining in the capsular bag **(Figure 11)**. Cohesive viscoelastic material is injected deep in the capsular bag to reform the bag and prepare it for IOL implantation. This helps to force the viscoelastic anteriorly facilitating its removal to prevent post-operative rise of IOP. [3]

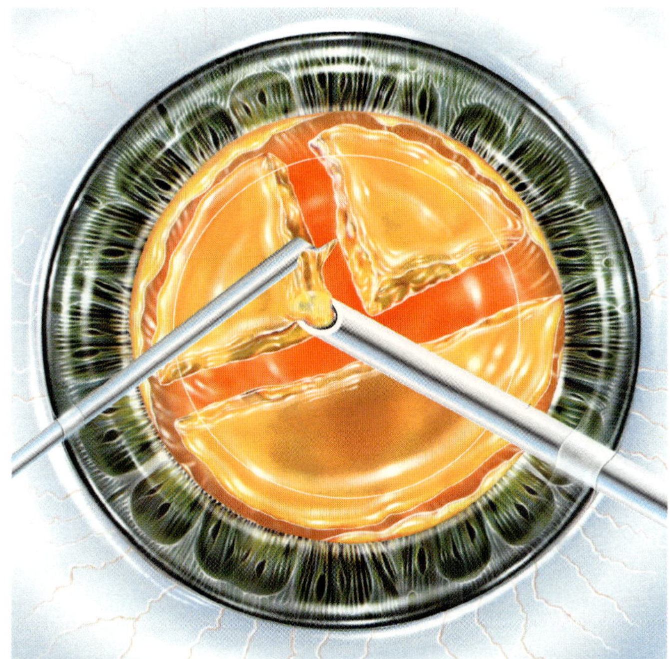

Figure 10: The 4 quadrants of the nucleus being emulsified during MICS surgery. (Art from Jaypee Highlights).

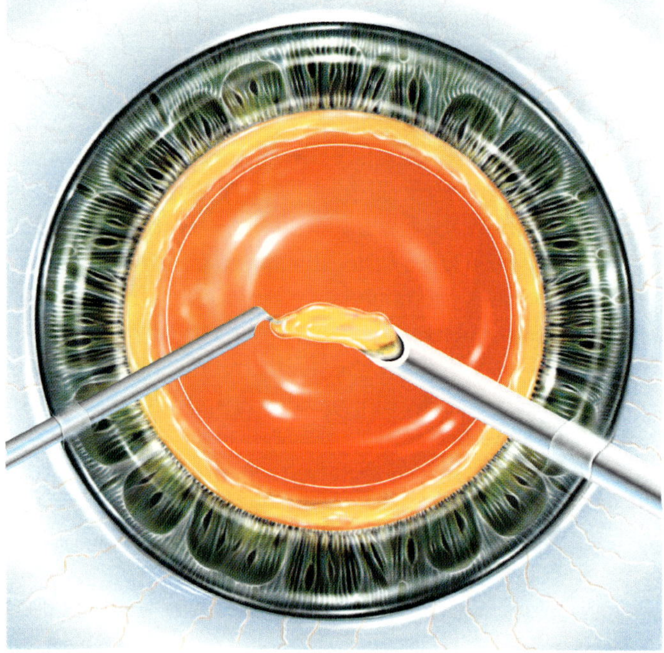

Figure 11: Bimanual cortex aspiration. (Art from Jaypee Highlights).

Results of LUS MICS

MICS surgery using ultrasound or laser, offers the advantage of having a superior biological effect on the ocular structures than conventional phaco procedures. Studying the parameters that control the procedure in both techniques the following was found:

Concerning the pressure of anterior chamber (AC), working in closed compartment through the microincisions, we found the pressure of AC to be higher in MICS surgery than in conventional phaco. Concerning the vacuum used during surgery it was found to be higher in MICS surgery, which is essential in performing this procedure. The average of ultrasound power differed according to the machine used. The grades of cataract operated with different machines were compared as illustrated. Less percentage of phaco was performed when using MICS burst 30 and 300 (Accurus system), but burst 300 mode offered less power delivered to the ocular tissue when the effective phaco time (EPT) was calculated **(Table 2)**.

Table 2: Comparison between the MICS and Phaco

	Phaco	MICS	P value
Mean cataract grade	3.05 (0.93 SD)	2.95 (0.99SD)	0.745
Mean incision size	3.3 (0.25 SD)	1.7 (0.21 SD)	0.001
Mean endothelial cell loss percentage	15.65 (19.96 SD)	11.37 (13.24 SD)	0.330
Mean flare value	12.37 (16.79 SD)	14.51 (17.01)	0.669
Mean ac cells	14.11 (17.59 SD)	11.2 (11.99 SD)	0.363
Mean phaco time	0.41 (0.44 SD)	0.38 (0.41 SD)	0.259
Mean power%	19.2 (10.98 SD)	5.28 (3.91 SD)	0.001
Mean EPT	9.2 (12.38 SD)	2.19 (2.77 SD)	0.001

Fluidics in MICS

In order to use the additional tool the flow of liquids must be fulfilled with the following conditions:

1. Stable incision with no leakage
2. Stable anterior chamber
3. High vacuum

When the diameter of the infusion cannulas is decreased a serious problem occurs. The anterior chamber does not start to fill up with the adequate amount of liquid. An infusion cannula diameter of 21 G is not able to maintain a stable anterior chamber at aspiration and under pressure of 500-600 mm Hg. Each attempt would end with the collapse of the anterior chamber.

Getting the high inflow of liquids into the anterior chamber is possible thanks to a new generation of tools. These tools have a relatively large infusion diameter and the right profile allowing the right flow of liquid and a low level of internal resistance. These conditions do not allow the anterior chamber to become shallow or rippling of the posterior capsule. Also, the correct amount of liquid ensures chilling of the phacoemulsification tip, and can function with highly efficient aspiration pumps.

According to laws of physics the interior diameter of the tool has a major influence on fluidic resistance, because resistance is proportional to the diameter.

Therefore, one is not allowed to apply standard infusion tools from the attention to the insufficient hydrodynamics of these units. Tools assuring the flow higher than 50 cc/min are needed for doing MICS. Current aspiration pumps have a utility which considerably exceeds the flow function of standard tools. The activity of standard infusion cannulas is estimated only for 30 cc/min.

Therefore the need for creating new tools arose in order to meet MICS needs. Katena Inc. (Denville, NJ, USA) took on the design and manufacture. A tool set came into existence with a very small diameter in answer to MICS requirements but at the same time with a high flow of about 72 cc/min.

Using the highly efficient pump we must allow the correct inflow of liquid into the anterior chamber. In the case of Accurus, Infinity type equipment we have the additional mechanism of pressurized inflow of fluidics - "gas forced infusion". This can allow controlling the increase in the pressure of the irrigation bottle. This mechanism pumps filtered gas into the irrigation bottle. It allows an additional increase in infusion. Highly efficient irrigation cannulas and the mechanism of gas forced infusion helps provide the comfort of working in stable anatomical conditions.

We can achieve anterior chamber stability in two ways. First, the high inflow of fluidics with proper instrument fluidics flow and forced infusion of fluidics. Secondly, reduced outflow. The diminished diameter of tools and the Cruise Control stable chamber system allow proper outflow without reducing the vacuum.

MICS can be done with different kinds of aspiration systems. However, a Venturi Pump system is most popular and recommended. It has great flexibility, fast reaction. It allows high value of under pressure and the flow as the additional important tool in breaking and removing masses of the lens. The flow can be adjusted, through the amount of vacuum and degree of occlusion of the tip. At present venturi is the most efficient system. MICS settings with different phacoemulsification platforms are shown in **Tables 3, 4 and 5**.

Astigmatism Control with MICS

Among the major advantages of MICS is the reduction of surgical trauma resulting in a reduction of surgically induced astigmatism (SIA), aberrations and improvement of the optical quality of the cornea after surgery, thus leading to improvement of visual outcome and high patient satisfaction.[9, 10]

Degraded optical quality of the cornea after incisional cataract surgery would limit the performance of the pseudophakic eye. Thus, it is important not to increase or to induce astigmatism and/or corneal aberrations after cataract surgery.[11] Even with MICS, we could achieve reduction of astigmatism and higher order corneal aberrations.[12] The optical quality of the cornea plays an important role in the recovery of the visual function after cataract surgery, and this is determined

Table 3: Accurus 600 Alcon settings for 19G MICS

Quad	Phacoemulsification Power	20%
	Vacuum	300 mm Hg
	Irrigation	90
	Mode burst	30 ms

Table 4: Infinity Alcon settings for 19G MICS

Chop	Phacoemulsification Power	0
	Dynamic rise	0
	Vacuum	150
	Irrigation	110
	Torsional amplitude	Limit:40
		On: 20
		Off: 40
	Aspiration rate	15
Quad	Phacoemulsification power	0
	Dynamic rise	2
	Vacuum	500
	Irrigation	110
	Torsional amplitude	Limit:80
		On: 20
		Off: 40
	Aspiration rate	30
Epi	Phacoemulsification power	0
	Vacuum	28
	Irrigation	110
	Torsional amplitude	Limit:80
		On: 20
		Off: 40
	Aspiration rate	28
Note: For 21 G MICS forced air infusion with air pump is necessary.		

Table 5: Millennium Bausch & Lomb settings for 19G MICS

Sculpture	Bottle height	100 cm
	Maximum bottle infusion	40 mm HG
	Fixed vacuum	200 mm HG
	Fixed U/S	10%
	Duration	20 ms
	Duty cycle	60%
Quadrant	Bottle height	100 cm
	Maximum bottle infusion	40 mm HG
	Fixed vacuum	470 mm HG
	Fixed U/S	10%
	Duration	20 ms
	Duty cycle	60%
I/A	Bottle height	80 cm
	Maximum bottle infusion	40 mm HG
	Fixed vacuum	550 mm HG
Note: For 21 G MICS forced air infusion with air pump is necessary.		

by a combination of corneal and internal aberrations generated by the IOL and those induced by the surgery. These corneal refractive changes are attributed to the location and size of the corneal incision. The smaller the incision, the lower the aberrations, the better the optical quality.[13]

We have described the improved control of surgically induced astigmatism with MICS when compared to conventional 3 mm phacoemulsification. A great advantage of MICS is the reduction of SIA and that the microincisions do not produce an increase in astigmatism.[14] The shorter the incision, the less the corneal astigmatism, as it was estimated that the magnitude of the SIA studied by vector analysis is around 0.44 and 0.88 diopters, rising as the size of the incision increases.[15,16] This is considered important because cataract surgery today is considered more and more a refractive procedure.[14]

Study of Endothelial Cell Count and Inflammatory Reaction

MICS surgery offers the advantage of lowering the percentage of cell loss during this procedure. Comparing the results of endothelial cell count pre and post-op there was no statistical significant difference between the numbers although the cell loss was reduced in MICS surgery. The flare and inflammatory cells developing after the procedure were found to be much lower in MICS surgery **(Table 6)**.

Table 6: Flare and Inflammatory Cell Reaction

		Conventional phaco (Mean ± SD)		MICS surgery (Mean ± SD)	
Pre-operative	Flare value	5.8	6.3	3.8	3.3
	Inflammatory cells	0.74	1.5	0.5	0.8
First month	Flare value	9.9	11.1	5.7	3.3
	Inflammatory cells	1.5	1.5	1.3	1.2
Third month	Flare value	5.2	3.5	5.2	2.3
	Inflammatory cells	0.9	1.1	0.6	0.5

Conclusions

MICS surgery is a popular technique in crystalline lens surgery. With the improved technology of phacoemulsificator machines and the power settings together with adequate instruments all the cataract grades are amenable to MICS. Refractive lens exchange using MICS technique has the advantage of preventing induced astigmatism and wound complications problems.

Editorial Comment

The main objective of the MICS is to perform small corneal incisions that produce the least surgically induced astigmatism possible. This provides better visual quality, less optical aberration and a greater patient satisfaction with the surgical results. The development of new instruments with small diameters that allow high inflow of fluids in the anterior chamber (of approximately 72 cc/min), the availability of surgical equipments that pressurize inflow of fluid into the eye by means of gas, as well as the Cruise Control devices that regulate the outflow of fluids, make this surgery nowadays a safe and effective procedure.

Arnaldo Espaillat, MD

References

1.	Shearing SP, Relyea RL, Loaiza and, Shearing RL. Routine phacoemulsification through a one millimeter non-sutured incision. Cataract 1985;2:6-11.
2.	Alió JL. What is the future of cataract surgery?. Ocular Surg News 2006;17:3-4.
3.	Alió JL, Rodriguez-Prats JL, Galal A: Micro-incision cataract surgery. Highlights of Ophthalomology International, Miami USA; 2004.
4.	Alió JL, Schimchak P, Montés-Micó R, Galal A. Retinal image quality after microincision intraocular lens implantation. J Cataract Refract Surg 2005;31:1557-60.
5.	Assaf A, El-Moatassem Kotb AM. Feasibility of bimanual microincision phacoemulsification in hard cataracts. Eye 2007;21:807-11.
6.	Tsuneoka H, Hayama A, Takahama M: Ultrasmall-incision bimanual phacoemulsification and AcrySof SA30AL implantation through a 2.2 mm incision. J Cataract Refract Surg. 2003 Jun; 29: 1070-6.
7.	Tsuneoka H, Shiba T, Takahashi Y. Ultrasonic phacoemulsification using a 1.4 mm incision: clinical results. J Cataract Refract Surg. 2002 Jan;28:81-6.
8.	Chylack, LT, Wolfe J K, Singer D M, et al: Lens opacities classification system III. Arch Ophthalmol 1993; 111:831-3.
9.	Alió JL, Rodriguez-Prats JL, Galal A. Advances in microincision cataract surgery intraocular lenses. Curr Opin Ophthalmol 2006;17:80–93.
10.	Naeser K, Knudsen EB, Hansen MK. Bivariate polar value analysis of surgically induced astigmatism. J Refract Surg 2002;18:72-78.
11.	Yao K, Tang X, Ye P. Corneal astigmatism, high order aberrations, and optical quality after cataract surgery: Microincision versus small-incision. J Refract Surg 2006;22: 1079-82.
12.	Jiang Y, Le Q, Yang J, Lu Y. Changes in corneal astigmatism and high order aberrations after clear corneal tunnel phacoemulsification guided by corneal topography. J Refract Surg 2006;22:1083-88.
13.	Holladay JT. Optical quality and refractive surgery. Int Ophthalmol Clin 2003;43:119-136.
14.	Alió JL, Rodriguez-Prats JL, Galal A, Ramzy M. Outcomes of microincision cataract surgery versus coaxial phacoemulsification. Ophthalmology 112:1997-2003.
15.	Vasavada AR, Singh R, Apple DJ, Trivedi RH, Pandey SK, Werner L. Effect of hydrodissection on intraoperative performance: Randomized study. J Cataract Refract Surg 2002;28:1623-28.
16.	Simsek S, Yasar T, Demirok A, Cinal A, Yilmaz OF. Effect of superior and temporal clear corneal incisions on astigmatism after sutureless phacoemulsification. J Cataract Refract Surg 1998;24:515-18.

<h1>7 | Microcoaxial and Torsional Phaco</h1>

Lincoln Lemes Freitas, MD
Flavio Koji Narazaki, MD

Introduction

First described in 1967, by Charles D. Kelman, lens extraction by phacoemulsification, had between its ideals to allow surgical procedure that promote rapid visual recovery, less damage to the intraocular structures and greater predictability of the final refractive results due to the smaller incision needed.[1-3] Passed over for almost 30 years, only in the early '90s, after the development of foldable intraocular lenses, this technique was rescued, achieving the status of gold standard for cataract surgery.[4-6]

Its objectives were maintained throughout these years and all current efforts aimed at the discovery of technologies that enable safer surgery with few complications, among them the development of torsional phacoemulsification and phacoemulsification through microincision, objects of this chapter.

Ultrasound Types

Practically all phacoemulsification machines use the piezoelectric properties of crystals for the production of the ultrasonic motion performed by the titanium tip attached to the handpiece, promoting the fragmentation of the lens. Since the first devices, vibration of the tip is directed longitudinally in a back-forward movement at a predetermined fixed frequency of 20-60KHz, depending on the manufacturer choice and allows adjusting the proportion of excursion of the tip

(Phaco Power) according to the surgeon's preference, promoting the emulsification of the lens by a "jackhammer" effect **(Figure 1)**.

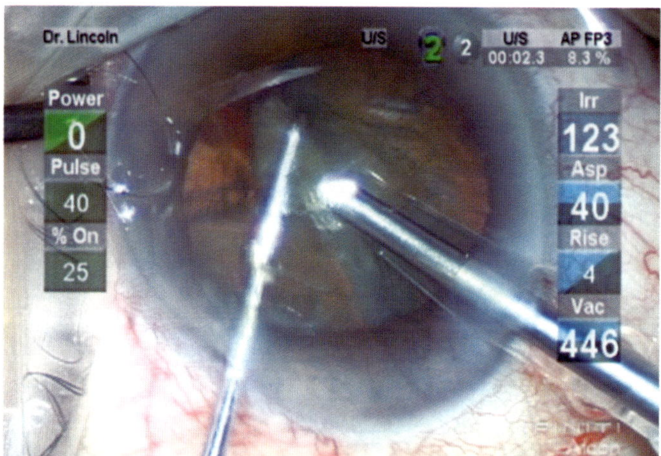

Figure 1: Cataract surgery using the longitudinal ultrasound.

At first ultrasonic vibration was activated continuously, causing a series of surgical complications related to the amount of energy released during the extraction of the lens, such as wound burn, corneal endothelial cell loss and subsequent development of bullous keratopathy.[7-13] Aiming to reduce the energy expended during the phacoemulsification were developed modulations of the firing of ultrasound, such as pulse mode, burst mode, micropulse mode and duty cycle control mode.

The pulsed mode is the earliest of these, it allows to determinate the number of pulses that are performed in one second, in each pulse the ultrasound is triggered at half the time and the other half the device only irrigates and aspirates, which cools the tip.

In the burst mode, it´s possible to choose the duration time of activation of ultrasound (time ON) in milliseconds, for a cycle of 2500 milliseconds, and as we move the footswitch, the time OFF decreases until the ultrasound becomes continuous.

With the micropulse mode you can work with pulses of only 4 milliseconds, which led to a drastic reduction of heat released, receiving the cold phaco denomination.[14-17] At the same time became possible to control the duty cycle, what means to determine the proportion of time to drive the ultrasound, which allows more time for cooling the tip, however this can extend the surgical time.

Despite these modulations of longitudinal phacoemulsification present satisfactory results for most of cataract surgeries, in cases of dense cataract or eyes with low endothelial cell count, we still observe high variability of surgical outcomes.

Seeking greater effectiveness in the use of ultrasonic energy to the cataract extraction surgery, in 2005, Alcon released to the market the Infiniti -Ozil® torsional phacoemulsification system, which applies a side-to-side oscillatory movement to fragmentation of the lens **(Figure 2)**.

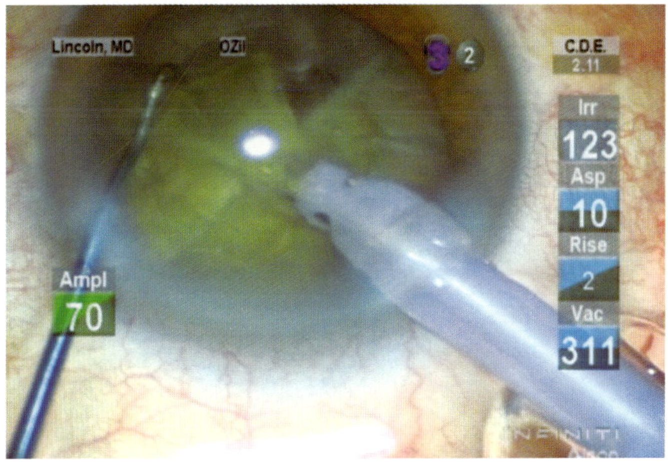

Figure 2: Cataract surgery using only the torsional ultrasound.

Working Method of the Torsional Ultrasound

Using crystals arranged transversally in the handpiece, the Ozil® system produces rotational movements at a frequency of 32KHz, which are transferred to a curved or angled tip, promoting the emulsification of the lens through the side-to-side oscillation performed by the tip. The torsional motion loses effect when using straight tip and earn greater amplitude with more angled tips, being the Kelman´s type tips the most indicated. You can achieve a range of motion of up to 2°, being determined by the angle of the tip and the surgeon's preference parameter.

It is possible to set the drive mode of ultrasound, including continuous, pulsed or burst, or customize the pulses, allowing more control of the energy released. The Infiniti-Ozil® system allows to combine the torsional technology with the longitudinal US, but the two types of ultrasound cannot work simultaneously, they are fired interchangeably **(Figure 3)**.

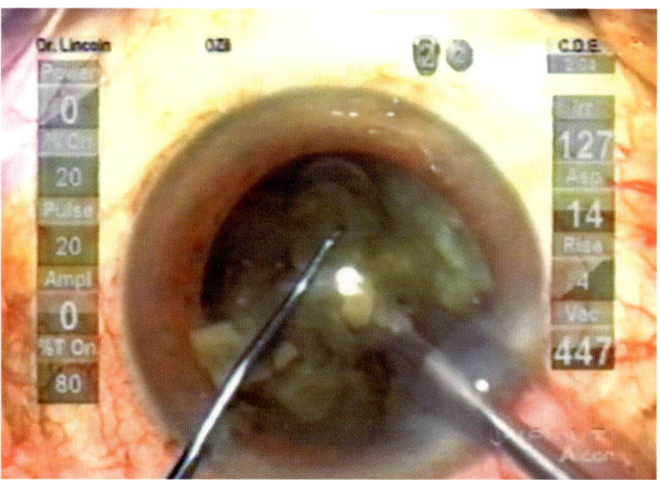

Figure 3: Cataract surgery using the torsional and longitudinal ultrasound.

Advantages and Drawbacks of Torsional Ultrasound

A remarkable feature of this technology is the reduction of energy waste during surgery by the lower frequency of ultrasound, 32KHz compared to 40KHz of most longitudinal ultrasounds, and to take better advantage on the lens fragmentation with the rotational movement.[18-20] The extremity of the tip remains in contact with the lens fragment the whole time, which does not happen in the longitudinal US because of its own characteristic movement that has a retrograde component, so only in 50% of the time the longitudinal US is actually fragmenting the lens.

The anterograde movement of the tip in longitudinal US can cause the repulsion of the lens, while the retrograde motion allows the loss of contact between the tip and the lens, favoring undesirable aspiration of other intraocular structures, such as the iris and the lens capsule, and occurrence of chattering, which can greatly compromise the surgical outcome. The absence of retrograde motion in the torsional phacoemulsification increases followability, and make these complications less frequent.[21,22]

Heat generation around incision observed in the torsional US is also a factor of great progress on this technology as a result of less energy used, and lower friction caused by rotational motion, producing temperatures a third of those reached by traditional US, is almost not observed wound burn, which reduces the risk of dehiscence, and endophthalmitis therefore[23,24] **(Figure 4).**

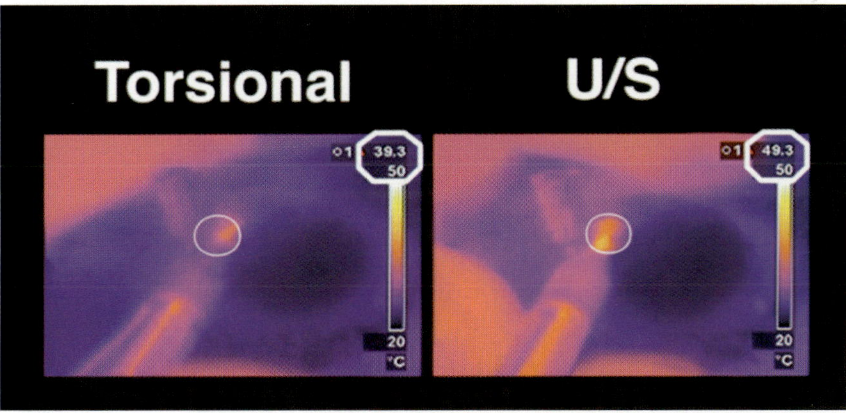

Figure 4: Temperature sensitive recording showing smaller temperatures using the torsional ultrasound during a cataract surgery.

The low energy released makes the torsional US ideal for sculpting sulcus, providing more security for surgeons who prefer the divide and conquer or the Stop and Chop techniques.

No changes are necessary in the parameters of irrigation, aspiration and vacuum, and the adaptation to an angled tip does not offer much difficulty, so virtually no learning curve in the transition from traditional to torsional phacoemulsification.

However this technology can work in an unsatisfactory way in some steps of surgery. By the torsional movement characteristics the tip is unable to produce cavitation of the lens and complete occlusion, which can theoretically difficult the adequate apprehension to perform the maneuvers of the Phaco Chop or Quick Chop techniques. It is not observed difficulty to penetrate the tip in the lens in practice.

In denser cataracts, was observed with relative frequency obstruction of the tip during surgery, when working exclusively with the torsional US. This inconvenience could be solved with the combination of the two types of ultrasound, for example 20msec of longitudinal US at 30-50% of power and 80msec torsional US at 100% of amplitude. To work around this problem, Alcon offers in 2009 the Ozil® Intelligent Phaco (Ozil® IP) upgrade which activates the longitudinal US when the vacuum reaches a predetermined value, preventing that obstruction of the tip occurs **(Figure 5)**.

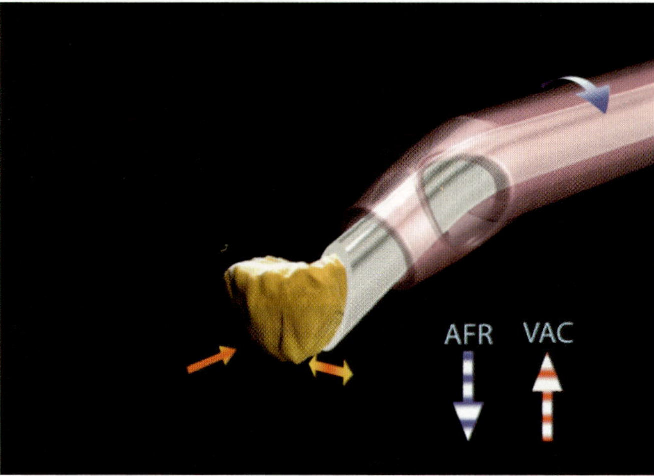

Figure 5: During the occlusion, the IP control system selects the best moment to release longitudinal ultrasound when the vaccum (VAC) is elevated. (AFR = aspiration).

With this modulation is possible to work always with the same parameters, independent of the cataract density, this should only be applied when using the torsional US exclusively during the removal of fragments, and it is not indicated for the lens fracture phases, because it disable the apprehension.

Unfortunately older devices cannot be adapted to this new technology, so it will take years for all countries to benefit from the advantages emanating from this new phacoemulsification method.

Microcoaxial Technology – Work Methods

The phacoemulsification technique and foldable lens implantation allowed a reduction of the incision size, from 12mm used in the intracapsular or extracapsular lens extraction techniques to 2.8 mm standard phacoemulsification, which reduced rates of serious surgical complications, as endophthalmitis and choroidal hemorrhages, and had enabled faster recovery of visual acuity, mainly due to lower induced astigmatism.[25-29] From this moment cataract surgery has acquired a concept more refractive and more surgeons engaged in developing technologies to smaller incisions.

MICS (Microincisional Cataract Surgery), a term first used by Jorge Alió, to denominate surgeries with 2mm incisions or smaller, which was realized with bimanual phacoemulsification technique of the lens.[30,31] The surgeon must build two incisions and work with irrigation separately from aspiration/phaco tip. The bimanual technique allowed incisions even smaller as Tsuneoka 1.4 mm, and 0.9 mm and 0.7 mm achieved by Agarwal, with the Phakonit and Microphakonit techniques respectively.[32-35] However, many surgeons have not adopted these techniques because of their variable learning curve, limitation of the lens manipulation and increase of surgical time for not impressive superior results to the standard phacoemulsification, besides the lack of IOLs with satisfactory quality for such a small incision.

Microcoaxial technology is another line of research for microincision surgeries. Through the development of silicon irrigation sleeves with smaller diameter associated with advanced mechanisms of fluidic control, it became possible to extract the lens with a very similar to standard phaco characteristics surgery by a 2.2 to 1.8 mm incision **(Figure 6)**.

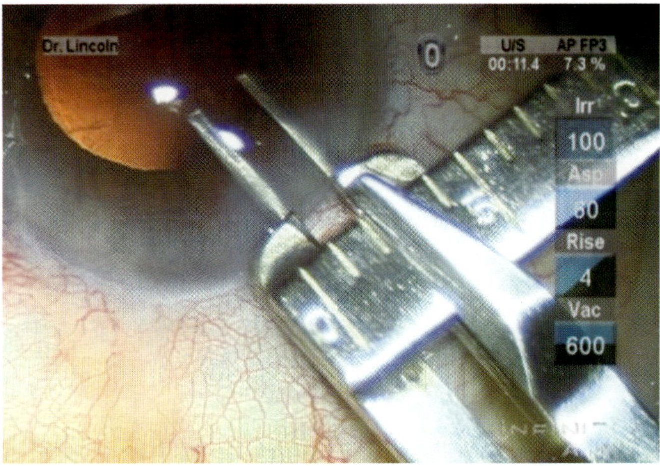

Figure 6: Cataract surgery using a 2.0mm clear cornea incision.

Modern silicon sleeves, as MicroSmoth Ultra® Alcon, have, in addition to the smaller diameter, thinner walls, ability to maintain satisfactory flow parameters for medium to high vacuum and also the ability to inflate across the wound, protecting corneoscleral tissue of the tip friction and reducing fluid loss through the incision, allowing more stable anterior chamber during surgery.

The best fluidic control introduced into modern phaco machines, especially the superior anti-surge mechanism, avoiding sudden decompression of the anterior chamber after the loss of occlusion of the tip, together with new technologies for better use of ultrasonic energy are also crucial for a safe microcoaxial surgery without complications that the lowest flow of infusion could cause, such as posterior capsule rupture and thermal injury to the incision.

Advantages and Drawbacks to Other Technologies

Compared to coaxial phacoemulsification, microcoaxial surgery presents, in light of the new designs of the silicon sleeve with soft-walled technology, best system of sealing the incision, which provides greater stability of the anterior chamber during surgery. This innovation does not cause loss of structural integrity of the wound, as seen in surgeries with more rigid sleeve or bimanual technique, where the steel is in direct contact with the walls of the wound, which has a negative impact in the incision closure at the end of surgery, increasing the risk of endophthalmitis.[36-43] In fact becomes even easier to seal it, requiring fewer stromal hydration.

There is practically no learning curve, maintaining usual technique of phaco-emulsification, just need to perform it with a smaller incision.[44] No need to change surgical instruments, even the capsulorhexis can be performed with the routine forceps, in contrast to bimanual technique that can promote a long learning curve, being necessary to readjust the confection of the capsulorhexis and manipulation of the lens, which becomes more complex.

The microcoaxial technology offers surgical procedure with rapid visual rehabilitation, minimal induced astigmatism and high visual quality, since it is already available on the market a wide range of foldable intraocular lenses capable of being injected into 2.2mm incisions, or less than 2.0mm when employing the countertraction implantation technique.[43,44,46] Maintaining the same quality and technological advancement of the best IOLs designed for standard coaxial phacoemulsification. As example we can mention: AcrySof single-piece IOL (Alcon Laboratories, Fort Worth, Texas), Idea 2.2 (Xcelens, Geneva, Switzerland), IOLTech MICS (IOLTech, La Rochelle, France), C-flex 570C (Rayner, East Sussex, UK), Akreos MI60 (Bausch & Lomb, Rochester, NY).

The restriction of the infusion rate of cataract phacoemulsification surgeries with microincision, about 35% less, requires to reduce the aspiration and vacuum parameters, reducing the advantages of fluidic dynamic, which slows the surgery and leads to an increase in the procedure time.[45,46] However, modern devices with better ultrasound modulation and better fluidic performance attempt to compensate this deficit **(Figure 7)**. In addition, theoretically, a lower flow in the anterior chamber decreases the damage to the corneal endothelial cells.

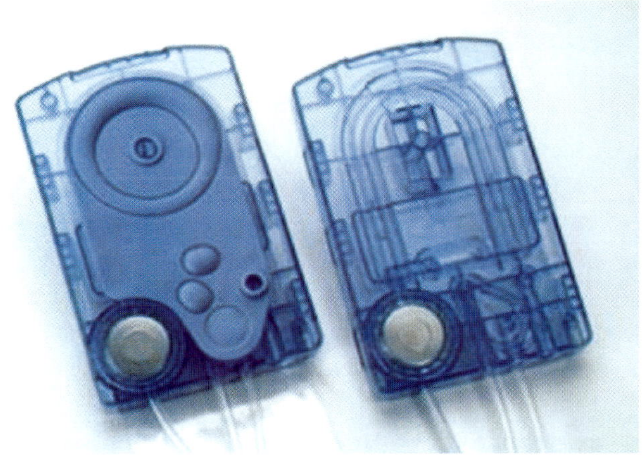

Figure 7: Intrepid system designed exclusively for microcoaxial cataract surgery.

Microcoaxial and Torsional

Alcon joined in INFINITI® Vision System properties of Ozil® torsional phacoemulsification with advances in microcoaxial technology, more specifically, developing the MicroSmoth Ultra® irrigation sleeve and INTREPID® Fluidic Management System. This combination offers the possibility of cataract surgeons perform a microincisional surgery with appropriate quality and safety by preventing the occurrence of chattering, increasing followability, decreasing risk of wound burns and surge.[19,24,42]

Discussion

Microincisional surgery is an important advance in cataract extraction and, with microcoaxial technology, can be assimilated without difficulty by an anterior segment surgeon accustomed to the traditional phacoemulsification. The undoubted improvements offered by the torsional ultrasound combined with microcoaxial adaptations facilitated greatly the transition process.

Even though it is a safe procedure, it is not indicated for all cases and should be reserved for the routine cataract. In difficult cases, it is prudent to choose performing the standard procedure due to the difficulties of manipulating the lens at very small incisions.

The surgical quality obtained with this technology allows us to believe that soon the majority of surgeons would probably be adopting microcoaxial surgery as standard procedure for cataract phacoemulsification.

Editorial Comment

After 2005 Alcon Laboratories' innovative Infiniti-Ozil® torsional phacoemulsification system for cataract surgery was introduced, meaning a great advance for varied reasons: delivering lower frequency ultrasonic energy and inducing only 2 degrees of torsional movement of the phaco needle, generate less friction against the incisional corneal tissue than the longitudinal phacoemulsification, thus reducing the risk of corneal burns. At the same time this fact allows small incision (2.2 to 2 mm) surgery, which induces a lower amount of astigmatism. Torsional movement does not induce repulse of the emulsified lens tissue, thus improving surgical followability and reducing the risk for endothelial damage. In order to prevent phaco tip obstruction by hard cataracts, Ozil® Intelligent Phaco (Ozil IP) upgrade was developed. The Intrepid fluid management system permits controlling the anterior chamber stability in cases of small incisions where a lower ocular inflow occurs compared with greater incisions. Working through small coaxial micro-incisions means that the surgical instruments do not have to be different from those that can be usually found in cataract surgery; the learning curve is negligible; and foldable, high technology intraocular lenses can be inserted (with aspherical optical surface, toric and multifocal lenses).

Arnaldo Espaillat, MD

References

1. Kelman CD. Phacoemulsification and aspiration. A new technique of cataract removal. A preliminary report. Am J Ophthalmol. 1967 Jul;64(1):23-35.
2. Kelman CD. Phaco-emulsification and aspiration. A progress report. Am J Ophthalmol. 1969 Apr;67(4):464-77.
3. Kelman CD. Phacoemulsification and aspiration. A report of 500 consecutive cases. Am J Ophthalmol. 1973 May;75(5):764-8
4. Leaming DV. Practice styles and preferences of ASCRS members – 1985 survey. J Cataract Refract Surg. 1986 Jul;12(4):380-4.
5. Leaming DV. Practice styles and preferences of ASCRS members – 1991 survey. J Cataract Refract Surg. 1992 Sep;18(5):460-9.
6. Leaming DV. Practice styles and preferences of ASCRS members – 1994 survey. J Cataract Refract Surg. 1995 Jul;21(4):378-85.
7. Werblin TP. Long-term endothelial cell loss following phacoemulsification: model for evaluating endothelial damage after intraocular surgery. Refract Corneal Surg. 1993 Jan-Feb;9(1):29-35.
8. Dick HB, Kohnen T, Jacobi FK, Jacobi KW. Long-term endothelial cell loss following phacoemulsification through a temporal clear corneal incision. J Cataract Refract Surg. 1996 Jan-Feb;22(1):63-71.
9. Díaz-Valle D, Benítez del Castillo Sánchez JM, Castillo A, Sayagués O, Moriche M. Endothelial damage with cataract surgery techniques. J Cataract Refract Surg. 1998 Jul;24(7):951-5.
10. Kohlhaas M, Klemm M, Kammann J, Richard G. Endothelial cell loss secondary to two different phacoemulsification techniques. Ophthalmic Surg Lasers. 1998 Nov;29(11):890-5.

11. Ernest P, Rhem M, McDermott M, Lavery K, Sensoli A. Phacoemulsification conditions resulting in thermal wound injury. J Cataract Refract Surg. 2001 Nov;27(11):1829-39.

12. Sippel KC, Pineda R Jr. Phacoemulsification and thermal wound injury. Semin Ophthalmol 2002 Sep-Dec;17(3-4):102-9.

13. Bradley MJ, Olson RJ. A survey about phacoemulsification incision thermal contraction incidence and causal relationships. Am J Ophthalmol. 2006 Jan;141(1):222-4.

14. Soscia W, Howard JG, Olson RJ. Microphacoemulsification with WhiteStar. A wound-temperature study. J Cataract Refract Surg. 2002 Jun;28(6):1044-6.

15. Donnenfeld ED, Olson RJ, Solomon R, Finger PT, Biser SA, Perry HD, Doshi S. Efficacy and wound-temperature gradient of whitestar phacoemulsification through a 1.2 mm incision. J Cataract Refract Surg. 2003 Jun;29(6):1097-100.

16. Olson RJ, Jin Y, Kefalopoulos G, Brinton J. Legacy AdvanTec and Sovereign WhiteStar: a wound temperature study. J Cataract Refract Surg. 2004 May;30(5):1109-13.

17. Fishkind W, Bakewell B, Donnenfeld ED, Rose AD, Watkins LA, Olson RJ. Comparative clinical trial of ultrasound phacoemulsification with and without the WhiteStar system. J Cataract Refract Surg. 2006 Jan;32(1):45-9.

18. Liu Y, Zeng M, Liu X, Luo L, Yuan Z, Xia Y, Zeng Y. Torsional mode versus conventional ultrasound mode phacoemulsification: randomized comparative clinical study. J Cataract Refract Surg. 2007 Feb;33(2):287-92.

19. Berdahl JP, Jun B, DeStafeno JJ, Kim T. Comparison of torsional handpiece through microincision versus standard clear corneal cataract wounds. J Cataract Refract Surg. 2008 Dec;34(12):2091-5.

20. Boukhny M. Laboratory performance comparison of torsional and conventional longitudinal phacoemulsification. Presented at: Annual Meeting of the American Society of Cataract and Refractive Surgery; March 17-22, 2006; San Francisco.

21. Solomon K. Performance of the Infiniti System: torsional vs conventional phacoemulsification handpieces. Presented at: Annual Meeting of the American Society of Cataract and Refractive Surgery; March 17-22, 2006; San Francisco.

22. Solomon K. Longitudinal vs torsional phacoemulsification. Presented as a sponsored booth presentation at: Annual Meeting of the American Society of Cataract and Refractive Surgery; March 17-22, 2006; San Francisco.

23. Han YK, Miller KM. Heat production: longitudinal versus torsional phacoemulsification. J Cataract Refract Surg. 2009 Oct;35(10):1799-805.

24. Jun B, Berdahl JP, Kim T. Thermal study of longitudinal and torsional ultrasound phacoemulsification: tracking the temperature of corneal surface, incision, and handpiece. J Cataract Refract Surg. 2010 May;36(5):832-7.

25. Watson A, Sunderraj P. Comparison of small-incision phacoemulsification with standard extracapsular cataract surgery: post-operative astigmatism and visual recovery. Eye (Lond). 1992;6 (Pt 6):626-9.

26. Cavallini GM, Lugli N, Campi L, Lazzerini A, Longanesi L. Surgically induced astigmatism after manual extracapsular cataract extraction or after phacoemulsification procedure. Eur J Ophthalmol. 1996 Sep;6(3):257-63.

27. Chee SP, Ti SE, Sivakumar M, Tan DT. Postoperative inflammation: extracapsular cataract extraction versus phacoemulsification. J Cataract Refract Surg. 1999 Sep;25(9):1280-5.

28. D Minassian, P Rosen, J Dart, A Reidy, P Desai, and M Sidhu. Extracapsular cataract extraction compared with small incision surgery by phacoemulsification: a randomized trial. Br J Ophthalmol. 2001 July; 85(7): 822–829.

29. Gogate PM, Kulkarni SR, Krishnaiah S, Deshpande RD, Joshi SA, Palimkar A, Deshpande MD. Safety and efficacy of phacoemulsification compared with manual small-incision cataract surgery by a randomized controlled clinical trial: six-week results. Ophthalmology. 2005 May;112(5):869-74.

30. Alió JL, Rodriguez-Prats JL, Galal A. MICS Micro-incision Cataract Surgery. Highlights of Ophthalmology International. El Dorado, Republic of Panama; 2004.

31. Alió J, Rodríguez-Prats JL, Galal A, Ramzy M. Outcomes of microincision cataract surgery versus coaxial phacoemulsification. Ophthalmology. 2005 Nov;112(11):1997-2003. Epub 2005 Sep 23.

32. Tsuneoka H, Shiba T, Takahashi Y. Feasibility of ultrasound cataract surgery with a 1.4 mm incision. J Cataract Refract Surg. 2001 Jun;27(6):934-40.

33. Tsuneoka H, Shiba T, Takahashi Y. Ultrasonic phacoemulsification using a 1.4 mm incision: clinical results. J Cataract Refract Surg. 2002 Jan;28(1):81-6.

34. Agarwal A, Agarwal A, Agarwal S, Narang P, Narang S. Phakonit: phacoemulsification through a 0.9 mm corneal incision. J Cataract Refract Surg. 2001 Oct;27(10):1548-52.

35. Agarwal A, Trivedi RH, Jacob S, Agarwal A, Agarwal S. Microphakonit: 700 micron cataract surgery. Clin Ophthalmol. 2007 Sep;1(3):323-5.

36. Vasavada AR. Phaco tips and corneal tissue: histomorphology and immunohistochemistry reveal the effects of sleeveless and sleeved tips. Cataract & Refractive Surgery Today. 2005 Jun(Suppl.):9-10.

37. Weikert MP, Koch DD. Phaco wound study: alterations in corneal wound architecture with bimanual microincisional phacoemulsification. Cataract & Refractive Surgery Today. 2005 Jun(Suppl.):11-13.

38. Berdahl JP, DeStafeno JJ, Kim T. Corneal wound architecture and integrity after phacoemulsification. Evaluation of coaxial micro incision and micro incision bimanual technique. J Cataract Refract Surg. 2007 Mar;33:510-515.

39. McDonnell PJ, Taban M, Sarayba M, Rao B, Zhang J, Schiffman R, Chen Z. Dynamic morphology of clear corneal cataract incisions. Ophthalmology. 2003 Dec;110(12):2342-8.

40. Gajjar D, Praveen MR, Vasavada AR, Pandita D, Vasavada VA, Patel DB, Johar K, Raj S. Ingress of bacterial inoculum into the anterior chamber after bimanual and microcoaxial phacoemulsification in rabbits. J Cataract Refract Surg. 2007 Dec;33(12):2129-34.

41. Johar S.R.K., Vasavada A.R., Praveen M.R., Pandita D., Nihalani B., Patel U., Vemuganti G. Histomorphological and immunofluorescence evaluation of bimanual and coaxial phacoemulsification incisions in rabbits. J Cataract and Refract Surg.2008 Apr;34(4):670-6.

42. Jun B, Berdahl JP, Kuo AN, Cummings TJ, Kim T. Corneal wound architecture and integrity after torsional and mixed phacoemulsification: evaluation of standard and microincisional coaxial techniques. Ophthalmic Surg Lasers Imaging. 2010 Jan-Feb;41(1):128-34.

43. Osher RH, Injev VP. Microcoaxial phacoemulsification Part 1: Laboratory studies. J Cataract Refract Surg. 2007 Mar;33(3):401-7.

44. Osher RH. Microcoaxial phacoemulsification Part 2: Clinical study. J Cataract Refract Surg. 2007 Mar;33:408-12.

45. Osher RH, Injev VP. Thermal study of bare tips with various system parameters and incision sizes. J Cataract Refract Surg. 2006 May;32:867-872.

46. Can I, Takmaz T, Yildiz Y, Bayhan HA, Soyugelen G, Bostanci B. Coaxial, microcoaxial, and biaxial microincision cataract surgery: prospective comparative study. J Cataract Refract Surg. 2010 May;36(5):740-6.

Index